The Low-Back Patient

Procedures for Treatment by Physical Therapy

Distributed by
YEAR BOOK MEDICAL PUBLISHERS · INC.
35 EAST WACKER DRIVE, CHICAGO

Joan G. LaFreniere, R.P.T.

Staff Physical Therapist
Department of Rehabilitation Medicine
New York Hospital at Cornell Medical Center
New York, New York

MASSON Publishing USA, Inc.
New York • Paris • Barcelona • Milan • Mexico City • Rio de Janeiro

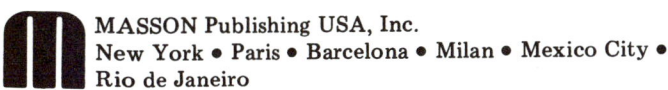

Dedication

This handbook was written as a contribution to the growth and development of the profession of Physical Therapy. It is dedicated to the many therapists who give unselfishly in both time and effort so that others may have a second chance at life . . . and living.

Third Printing, June, 1985

Copyright © 1979, by Masson Publishing USA, Inc.

All rights reserved. No part of this book may be reproduced in any form, by photostat, microform, retrieval system, or any other means, without the prior written permission of the publisher.

ISBN 0-89352-033-0
Library of Congress Catalog Card Number: 78-61474

Printed in the United States of America

Foreword

The author gives an account of her personal experience in the treatment of patients who suffer from low-back pain. She points out that there is no substitute for a detailed, careful evaluation of the low-back sufferer and for the application of a rational exercise program. The exercise program the author describes is based on sound physiological and kinesiological principles.

The value of the book is in its description of the careful guidance a patient with chronic low-back pain needs. The book will be of great value to those whose professional activities expose them to the treatment of low-back sufferers.

                      Willibald Nagler, M.D., F.A.C.P.
                      Chief, Rehabilitation Medicine
                      The New York Hospital-Cornell
                      Medical Center

Preface

This volume is a guide for physicians (especially physiatrists), hospital administrators, physical and occupational therapists, teachers, and patients.

The private physician who treats patients with low-back pain without the assistance of a physical therapist will find the evaluation worksheets useful in organizing all pertinent signs, symptoms, and clinical measurements. He or she is presented with a successful method of treating acute muscle spasm, and one which the patient can perform safely at home as a follow-up treatment. Handouts explaining ice therapy, exercise rationale, and instructions are included for the convenience of both the physician and the patient. From the bank of therapeutic exercises the physician can construct an individualized program to correct deficiencies for each patient dependent on the evaluation. Activities of daily living using correct body posture, movement, and mechanics, as well as information on conditioning the low-back patient for athletic activities, are also presented.

To the hospital administrator and/or physiatrist this book presents a complete, systematic approach to the treatment and management of the low-back patient. It offers all of the components necessary for instituting a successful method of treatment in a hospital setting, including the responsibilities of the physician and of the physical and occupational therapists in the treatment of the low-back patient. Evaluation worksheets, handouts for the education of the patient, and a complete bank of therapeutic exercises including relaxation techniques are included, together with the theory of application. A total approach to rehabilitating the low-back patient to a complete, satisfying life-style is presented in a manner that is applicable in a hospital setting because it is organized, with well-defined roles. Furthermore, this approach utilizes both personnel and facilities in a most efficient manner, which is important to both the patient and the hospital administration because that facilitates quality care.

To physical therapists this book is truly a handbook of "Physical Therapy Procedures for Treatment of the Low-Back Patient," because it deals solely with conservative, nonsurgical treatments within the realm of the physical therapist. Moreover, its logical, progressive-type approach to pain and musculoskeletal disorders of the back offers an alternative to the patient who would otherwise consider only surgery for pain-relief and/or an increase in functional activities. The physical therapist is presented with the components necessary for astute insight into the musculoskeletal kinesis of the back and concurrent pathologies most often found in clinical practice. This volume outlines the skills necessary to treat disorders of function that severely limit the activities of the patient and offers the physical therapist a truly professional approach to the treatment of the low-back patient, whether it be in the hospital setting or in private practice.

The occupational therapist has much to offer the low-back patient. The most important contributions, and the ones outlined in this text, are the teaching of daily living activities incorporating good body mechanics and the reinforcement of the proper attitudes necessary for readjustment to a functional lifestyle. These can be either preventive or rehabilitative measures, depending on the status of the patient. In these ways the occupational therapist can complement the efforts of the physical therapist by reinforcing good posture, movement, alignment, and body mechanics with a carry-over into functional activities.

To teachers in programs of physical therapy, physical therapy assistants, occupational therapists, nurses, and others in the allied health fields, this handbook offers itself as an organized course outline in the treatment of low-back pain. It is based on solid physiological theory and describes in detail a comprehensive evaluative procedure on which to base the treatment plan. All components of the proposed treatment plan are included and illustrated. Psychological considerations, and transfer techniques for patients in pain are also detailed. Each exercise group presented has many progressions, which means that there is room in this program "for the patient to progress." It is a program of satisfaction for both the therapist and the patient.

The advantages to students are many, the most important being that they will be graduating from their professional programs with more than a hot-pack and five standard exercises to offer their patients with low-back pain. This handbook is complete in theory, evaluation, treatment/management, conditioning, prevention, pain-control, modality-application, and other information necessary for an intelligent, professional approach to low-back pain.

To the patients, themselves, this volume is useful to help them obtain a deeper understanding of what causes their low-back pain. They can use the illustrated exercises while performing their daily exercise routine. Whether the patient is in an acute, management, or functional phase of rehabilitation or prevention, he or she can find information and guidance in this handbook.

Acknowledgments

To Christine E. Rath, R.P.T., Acting Chief of Physical Therapy at New York Hospital, for her patience in dealing with me, which on many occasions far surpassed human endurance levels . . . and for the time and energy she spent editing the original manuscript. A special "thank you."

To Dr. Hans Kraus who allowed me the opportunity to study with him.

To Dr. Willibald Nagler, Chief of Rehabilitation Services at New York Hospital, for his assistance and support in this effort.

To Dr. Ronald Green whose open-mindedness opened many doors for me.

To Ms. Joy Cordery, Coordinator of Rehabilitation Services at New York Hospital, for her cooperation.

To Susan Bergholtz . . . hail to the new Chief!

To the instructors at Columbia University School of Physical Therapy who gave me my basic education in Physical Therapy, especially Ms. Althea Jones.

To Lynn B. McDowell, MA, who contributed the illustrations contained herein.

To Regina Krug, a friend and professional, who many times steered me in the right direction when I got lost.

To Dana Stuart-Bullock, my friend and peer.

To Viera Novak . . . A physical therapist who is also an "irreplaceable person."

To the staff physical therapists, past and present, at New York Hospital for their invaluable contributions to our "back program," many times given by the "sweat of their brow" and with their "last ounce of energy," especially Patty Kozerefski, Eleanor Panzarino, Clara Neuman, Donna Cass, Amy Casden, and Jackie Schuyler.

To Isabel, Laura and Helen, and especially Rosemary Goldstein, who keep the books straight at New York Hospital.

To Judy and Linda who man the telephones, and keep us all straight.

To Vera and Blanca, for doing their jobs so well.

To Vera in Occupational Therapy . . . for being the special person that she is.

To the many patients at New York Hospital who have worked so diligently to regain their dignity and rightful place in society.

To G.L.H. . . . a truly unique individual, for contributing so much to my growth, both personally and professionally.

Contents

Foreword—W. Nagler, M.D.	iii
Preface	iv
Acknowledgments	vi
Chapter 1: The Personality Profile of the Low-Back Patient	1
Chapter 2: Anatomical Entities Relating to Low-Back Pain	29
Chapter 3: Evaluation: Doctor/Physical Therapist	42
Chapter 4: A Complete Low-Back Exercise Program	66
Chapter 5: Treatment/Management of the Low-Back Patient	133
Chapter 6: Body Movement and Mechanics	164
Index	192

Chapter 1

The Personality Profile of the Low-Back Patient

INTRODUCTION

As physical therapists we have all experienced the patient who refuses to "get better." Despite exhaustive diagnostic tests and extensive periods of therapy, some patients continue to live their lives as chronic low-back-pain sufferers. On the other hand, many of the patients treated for low-back pain at New York Hospital are treated for an "acute" episode only, and then are discharged with a preventative exercise program. A number of these will return sometime in the future for treatment of other "acute" episodes. But a high percentage of the low-back population respond favorably to an effective physical therapy regime for treatment of muscle spasm, triggerpoints, etc. (as detailed in Chapter 5), and continue to function in all aspects of their lifestyle, except during the initial onset of pain. The physical therapist derives immediate satisfaction from treating this segment of the low-back population, because of this favorable response to treatment and their immediate return to a functional capacity. It is the patient population with chronic low-back pain that causes frustration and confusion to the patients themselves and to the therapist.

It is evident to most who treat low-back patients for any length of time that an emotional component is either present at the time of the "acute" onset of pain or develops at some time thereafter. Many therapists complain that they are not psychiatrists or psychologists, and, therefore, should not be expected to treat patients who are emotionally disturbed or those whose pain is of a psychosomatic origin. While it is true that the physical therapist should not be the primary-care professional, the therapist has both an obligation and a specific role in the treatment of disabling, chronic low-back pain whether or not a specific abnormality is found.

There are three reasons for making this statement:

(1) The number of cases of back pain has reached epidemic proportions in our society. It is estimated that 80% of the general population will experience back pain in their lifetime, that low-back pain is the most expensive ailment in the 30 to 60 age group, that the yearly incidence is about 50 per 1,000 workers, and that the number of workdays lost is 1.400 per 1,000 American workers (Nachemson, 1976). Russek (1955) found that low-back pain accounted for 12.4% of industrial injuries and 16% of the compensation paid in New York State. More important is the implication, through extrapolation, that our national cost in 1974 for hospital-treated back problems was probably about $1.38 billion. This amount represents 1.4% of all dollars expended for health care in the United States in 1974 (Pheasant, 1977).

(2) The fact that other subspecialities do not devote either the time or the effort, nor do they have the interest necessary, for effective treatment of low-back pain. Approximately 1 million practitioners with varying backgrounds will treat a projected 2 billion patients (worldwide) suffering from low-back pain during the next decade. Only 500 physicians will try to evaluate their methods in a scientific way. There are probably no more than 50 scientists in the world today at work on elucidating the cause of our most expensive disease (Nachemson, 1976).

(3) Physical therapists are well qualified and in an ideal position to offer a professional approach for the relief of pain in the treatment of low-back patients. Their educational background in the necessary areas of anatomy, especially neurology, is more than adequate to gain an understanding of pain concepts. Furthermore, since pain is most times the most immediate presenting symptom and can often interfere with the treatment of choice, the therapist must deal with the patient's pain daily, and on a continuous basis. Pain relief/control is another service within the realm of Rehabilitation Medicine that could be rewarding for both the therapist and the patient.

This chapter will explore the dichotomy (acute vs. chronic) of the low-back-patient population, and explain the relationship between the personality processes and pain of a psychosomatic origin. The therapist's role in attempting to interrupt the "chain-of-events" that could produce a "chronic sufferer" will be discussed. Clinical signs of depression, conversion hysteria, and dependency will also be presented. The psychosomatic aspect of low-back pain will render the most effective physical therapy treatment *ineffective*. Through a personality profile and other precipitating factors, this chapter will examine underlying emotional processes which predispose an individual to a pattern of chronicity.

THE "ACUTE" PATIENT

Many physical therapy practices and hospital departments are dominated by the treatment of low-back patients. Approximately 50% of them are classified as patients with back pain of a traumatic origin and are referred to as patient's suffering from an "acute" episode. This is the "come-and-go" patient. They present typically with local pain, muscle spasm, and decreased functional activities. Their treatment is of a short duration and usually is successful. With intensive out-patient physical therapy, follow-up treatment at home, and guidance in body mechanics and ADL, the patient returns to normal functional activities after a few weeks. He continues on a preventive program of exercise indefinitely. Periodically, though, because of increased stress, strain or sprain, muscle weakness, or triggerpoints, one-half of this percentile will return for a short course of treatment. Should the patient return more than three times in a year, or experience a longer-lasting episode of low-back pain that severely interferes with functional activities (sleeping, sitting and standing, walking, bending, riding and driving in an automobile, and social and occupational responsibilities), he is considered to be progressing toward a "chronic low-back condition."

This is a crucial time in the treatment of the patient. It is a "signal" to the therapist that additional physical and/or psychological pathology is beginning to emerge. When a patient becomes excessively dependent on physical therapy treatment and/or his low-back pain interferes with normal functions, the therapist must look deeper into conditions surrounding the patient at that time. Are there problems at home, at work, or with interpersonal relationships? Has the patient felt an increase in anxiety or tension? At times some patients will be reluctant to divulge personal information. An effective way to approach this situation would be to ask the patient to trace his activities from the time of his last treatment to the present using the rationale that it is an attempt to find what activities might have caused the exacerbation.

Should the patient mention an individual in the course of his response, draw the person into the conversation by asking a very general question, such as, "Is he a friend?" or "Do you and your wife enjoy the same hobbies?" Do not act shocked, overly surprised, or condescendingly at anything the patient may reveal to you. At this time the patient needs a mature listener that he can trust with his thoughts and feelings. Let the patient know that his welfare is as important to you as it is to him. Show the patient that you care; it is the most effective way to develop a patient-therapist rapport. At times it could cause a turning point in the patient's life, as in the following example:

Example

Mrs. M. was a 65-year-old widow who came to the hospital because of pain in the right rhomboid. It kept her awake at night and ROM of the scapula was painful. The physician made an initial diagnosis of a triggerpoint in that muscle. Mrs. M. was put on a conservative treatment of electrical stimulation, friction massage, and exercise to stretch the muscle. She was status-post right mastectomy and cataract surgery. She ambulated with a cane and had difficulty with her vision.

After three weeks in therapy the therapist found Mrs. M. to be a warm, sensitive, and extremely religious woman. She was always cheerful when she arrived and had a story to tell about her faith in people and the "goodness" they showed toward her and others. The patient showed some progress from the treatments, but insisted that the pain was still intensive enough to warrant treatment.

At this time she requested an injection to dissolve the triggerpoint, and during post-triggerpoint injection therapy she talked extensively about her inability to see and the difficulties she was experiencing in coordinating her many medical appointments. It was suggested that she decrease her daily physical therapy appointments, but she quickly declined that suggestion. Mrs. M. talked frequently about her daughter who lived in California, whom she saw only a few times a year, and how much she missed her.

Following a period of relative calm, suddenly Mrs. M. arrived for therapy in a disheveled state for two consecutive days. On this particular day she had a flushed face, and was very tense. She had difficulty settling down enough to receive her treatment (since changed to microwave, massage, and exercise, as she was well into the second month of therapy). When questioned, Mrs. M. stated that she had four different doctors and when she really needed one last night, because she feared her blood pressure was up, she could not reach any of them. She had not felt well since the night before and couldn't sleep. She had several other appointments scheduled with different physicians for miscellaneous disorders. In addition, she felt she could not cope with the pain from her upper back, which by this time had also extended to the low-back area. She mentioned the Thanksgiving holiday, which was coming up at the end of the week, several times during the conversation.

The therapist did not have to be a psychiatrist to see that Mrs. M. could no longer cope with daily activities because of her failing eyesight compounded by increased loneliness and depression. This was exaggerated by the upcoming holiday.

Instead of beginning her usual treatment, the therapist took Mrs. M.'s blood-pressure and reassured her that it was within normal limits. Mrs. M.'s physician within the department was notified and asked for the name of an internist in the patient's neighborhood who could see to all of her medical needs. The physician was requested to call and make Mrs. M. an appointment, which he did. The patient was also informed of senior citizen groups in her area, and Lighthouse services for the blind. She was encouraged to talk about her daughter in California, and her frustration at the distance between them.

Mrs. M. returned two more times. Each time she revealed that her life was less complicated. She had visited her "new" doctor, and he regulated her blood-pressure medication, checked her other aches and pains, and reassured her that she was in relatively good health. She said that she was planning a trip to visit her daughter in California. Her new glasses had arrived and she could "see" a little bit better.

Mrs. M. said that her pain had decreased, she felt it only occasionally during certain movements and it no longer woke her at night. Since the stressful situations were lessened for her, she was more in control of her environment. She returned two more times, and then asked to be discharged from therapy. She left in good spirits and did not return.

Therapy in Mrs. M.'s case was not only physical therapy. It was supportive therapy. In her daughter's absence, someone had to care enough to help uncomplicate her life. Had her unbearable stress continued, she might have experienced a physical and/or emotional catastrophe. Since a very definite need for pain did exist in Mrs. M.'s case, she could have easily become a "Chronic Low-Back Sufferer."

THE "CHRONIC" PATIENT

The intervention of the therapist at appropriate times during treatment of the low-back patient cannot be overly stressed. The concept of treating the "total" patient must be realized continually, regardless of the length of treatment time, as many times this intervention will delay or even prevent a patient from progressing through the dynamic process shown in Figure 1. This schematic presentation illustrates the complexity of the relationship between personality processes and pain of a psychosomatic origin, which dominates the remaining 50% of back patients.

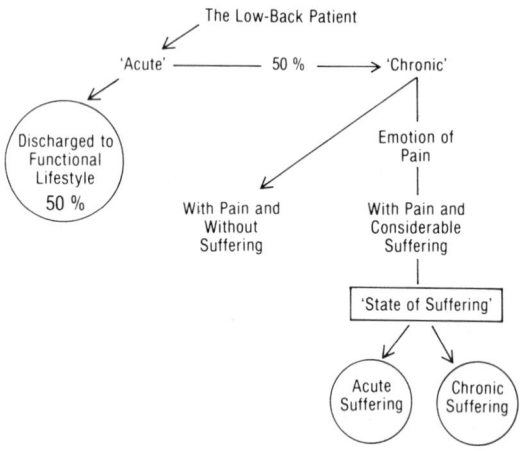

Figure 1. The dichotomy of the low-back-patient population explaining the relationship between personality processes and the chronicity of pain.

Note that all patients begin their low-back experience as an "acute" patient. The history (Sarno, 1976) of many of these patients begins with an episode that is somatic, such as severe back strain, sprain, contusion from trauma, or intervertebral disc pathology, at which time they are still considered to be in the acute state. Gentry and co-workers (1972) noted that 85% of the chronic low-back patients they studied could pinpoint a definite precipitating event to their pain, which included falling (20%), lifting or pushing objects such as batteries and lawnmowers (40%), traffic accidents (17%), and childbirth (8%). What is it, then, that causes 50% of the acute patients to be successfully treated in the acute stage and 50% to remain as patients and assume a more disabling role as the chronic low-back patient?

Figure 2 demonstrates two models constructed from data compiled from recent studies dealing with chronic back pain and psychic conflict (Tinling and Klein, 1966; Raskind and Mead, 1967; Gentry et al., 1972; Kolb, 1973; Wilson el al., 1974; Cairns et al., 1976; Nachemson, 1976; Mane, 1977). The psychological aspects affecting the pain-prone patient have been examined in extensive detail in controlled environments, such as in the rehabilitation setting at the Institute of Rehabilitation Medicine, at New York University Medical Center, New York City. These studies lend insight into the relationship between the psychogenic and the physiological aspects of chronic low-back pain.

a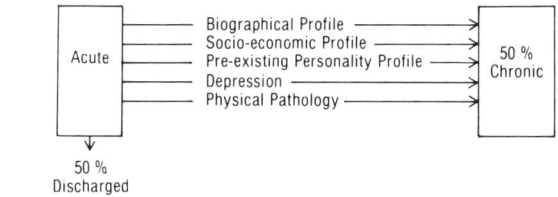

b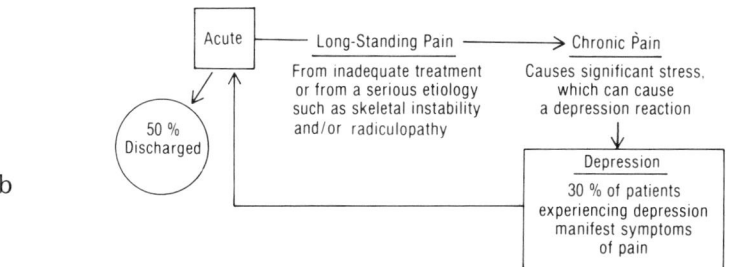

Figure 2. "Cause-and-effect" relationship between depression and chronic low-back pain.

As the physical therapist is treating a patient who is experiencing an "acute" episode of low-back pain and/or trauma, he must be aware of the following five precipitating factors that could predispose the patient to becoming a chronic sufferer often referred to as the "Low-Back Derelict" (Raskind and Mead, 1967):

    Biographical Profile

    Socioeconomic Profile

Preexisting Personality Profile

Depression

Physical Pathology (known or unknown)

Realistically, it is not always possible to extrapolate and compile all of the data necessary to complete, for example, a preexisting personality profile. This is true because of time limitations and/or lack of records, and psychiatric consults, etc. But for the problem patient, the one who "sends signals" exposing his or her existing emotional conflict or personality problems, the therapist should feel a professional obligation to spend time and effort in attempting to interrupt the chain-of-events that could produce a "chronic sufferer." This is preventive medicine, equal to teaching breathing exercises to a presurgical candidate, for example, and should receive appropriate emphasis in the therapists's time and effort expenditure.

From intensive investigation of chronic low-back patients, the emergence of the following profiles are presented. They broadly characterize the patient who suffers with severe, intractible, disabling back pain for which no specific abnormality is found, and are presented only to alert the therapist to additional descriptive "signs" of patients who have the propensity to chronicity.

Biological Profile (Gentry et al., 1972; Cairns et al., 1976)

The potential chronic low-back patient

- has an initial onset of symptoms at a relatively young age; 30.6 for females, 35.7 for males, 33.5 average;

- attributes his or her symptoms to a wide variety of minor causes, usually sprains, strains, or other minor trauma;

- tends to have less formal education: 11.7 years formal education for females, 10 years formal education for males, 10.8 average;

- begins work at an early age; 20 years old for females, 14.5 years old for males, 16 average;

- tends to be later-born child with many siblings;

- places an emphasis on family togetherness and interaction;

- may have had model figures who experienced chronic low-back pain that was unresponsive to conventional treatment (23% do).

Socioeconomic Profile (Gentry *et al.*, 1972; Cairns *et al.*, 1976)

The chronic low-back patient

- most were married at the onset of pain (98%);

- most had some form of compensation available at the time of initial onset;

- most had a stable work history: Average length of time at job at onset of initial symptoms was 7.2 years, and on the average patients held only two previous jobs;

- tended to be employed in jobs that required physically strenuous or overly routinized responsibilities;

- tended to work at blue collar manual or white collar clerical-type jobs (64%), to be housewives (18%), or to be professionals (11%);

- 59% tended to have a life experience including familial models for pain and/or major disability;

- often experienced little satisfaction from their jobs;

- often were a drug and/or alcohol abuser.

Preexisting Personality Profile

At the time a patient experiences an "acute" episode of low-back pain, any of the following psychic states or conflicts may already be present or emerge under the added stress:

Anxiety

Depression

Conversion hysteria

Masochism

Pain and loss

Strong dependency needs

The "need" for pain

It is important for the therapist to recognize the fact that the patient may be experiencing one of these manifestations as detailed below. At a time of an "acute" exacerbation the physical symptoms are the prevailing ones, and so dominate their mental source that they are not superficially recognizable. The patient rarely complains of his anxiety, depression, resentment, or sexual tension, but rather of his disorder of bodily function, such as anorexia, vomiting, backache, headache, or palpitation (Kolb, 1973).

The therapist might be tempted to switch the patient from treatment to treatment and finally discharge the patient as hopeless if he or she does not improve. Even if the patient is kept on program for an extended time when no methods of treatment seem successful, the therapists's attitude may be one of disinterest and hopelessness, which might be dangerous to the patient. This type of attitude might slowly edge him into the role of the chronic low-back patient, because he would not receive either the support and/or proper referral he so desperately needs from the therapist. If, on the other hand, the patient is discharged sooner, after several treatments fail, he will become a "low-back transient" and move from hospital to hospital, from therapist to therapist finding a similar situation with each.

Again, these are both situations in which the patient could easily be pushed into a chronic state, and from there, become a chronic sufferer, as illustrated in Fig. 2b.

Anxiety

Anxiety is a persistent feeling of dread, apprehension, and impending disaster. It is a response to threats from repressed dangerous impulses deep within the personality or to repressed feeling striving for consciousness, a warning of danger from the pressure of unacceptable internal attitudes. It differs from fear in not being referable to specific objects or events. The patient is ignorant of its source. Anxiety together with the various defensive mechanisms such as repression, regression, conversion, and displacement, constitutes an important factor in the psychopathology of abnormal personalities, psychoneurosis, psychoses, and psychosomatic disease (Kolb, 1973).

A patient will express a psychosomatic symptom when appropriate defenses breakdown and are failing to contain underlying conflict. This symptom prevents the patient from being overwhelmed by his anxiety, which explains why he often has an unconscious resistance to "letting go" of this defensive measure (the symptom).

Most patients treated at New York Hospital for low-back pain suffer from varying levels of anxiety as does most of the general population. For patients with mild anxiety, both general and local relaxation (pp. 77, 79) are stressed as an adjunct to his regular exercise program. In addition, the patient is offered emotional support in an atmosphere where he is encouraged to talk about stressful situations at home, at work, and in social situations. When a patient experiences more intense anxiety, the above methods should be more pronounced in the treatment plan; as Kolb emphasizes, if an emotional disorder is misidentified and mistreated as an organic disease, the patient's symptoms tend to become more chronic instead of improving. If the patient's anxiety becomes fixed on a somatic symptom, or if he believes that all of his troubles stem from an organic basis, successful treatment will be even more complicated.

Example

   Mrs. S. was 23 years old. She was a tall, attractive woman who had recently been married. Her chief complaint was pain in the left buttock. The diagnosis was unspecific, roentgenograms were normal, ROM was WNL. There was a slight decrease in MS in the left abductor. Her treatment was heat, electric stimulation, and mild strengthening exercises to the low back and left hip. The plan of treatment was to decrease pain and increase muscle strength. The goal was to return the patient to a full-functioning capacity.

   Mrs. S. related that her social, work, and home activities were limited because of the intense pain in her left buttock. She remained on program for a period of 3 to 4 weeks, and experienced varying levels of progress, then acute exacerbations. Intermittently, she received triggerpoint injections when triggerpoints were found to be the source of local pain. Each time the pain returned.

   Whenever the patient returned for treatment she concentrated completely on her somatic symptoms, relating the intensity of the pain in a shaky, emotional voice. She was almost always close to tears. She kept saying, "If only I could get rid of this pain, everything would be all right." She also mentioned that her husband was beginning to get intolerant of her sickness and pain, and was reluctant to invest anymore time or money into her treatment.

   At that time the patient requested a mild tranquilizer from the physician, which was granted. Finally the therapist decided that the emotional component of the pain the patient was experiencing was probably more dominant than anyone had originally suspected. This did not, however, rule out the search for other possible physical or mechanical causes as being a concomitant etiological factor of her pain. The patient did present also with a mild scoliotic curve, with a dominant thoracic and a compensating lordotic curve.

Since the treatment of the low-back and hip pain was not successful, the therapist switched the emphasis of the treatment on the upper back and correction of the scoliosis. Since the patient occasionally felt "fatigue" pain and strain in that area, she was put on a program of breathing and relaxation exercises, heat, and several exercises to correct the abnormal scoliotic curves. The patient "felt much better" for about 1 week on this program, but then totally regressed. The pain in her left buttock increased, and eventually she felt excruciating pain across the upper back. The patient called on the phone, hysterically, and related her new symptoms. She was told to stop all exercises until her next physical therapy appointment. Her physician was notified and he knew of no organic cause for her pain.

The patient returned in a very emotional state, saying, "I don't know what I'm going to do ... nothing works ... if only the pain would go away ... " During a treatment of relaxation exercises, it was suggested to the patient that she receive some help from a psychiatrist as an accompaniment to physical therapy treatment. She defended the position that all of the problems she was experiencing at home arose from her physical symptoms, and that if she could cure the pain, the other problems would disappear. So, why should she see a psychiatrist? The therapist pointed out that in some instances emotional stress intensifies physical problems, and it was difficult in her case to get to the "root" of her problem when she was so upset. She agreed, but said that her husband wouldn't pay for any further treatments and that they couldn't afford it, anyway. She insisted, however, in continuing with physical therapy treatments.

As the therapist was investigating what psychiatric services were available to Mrs. S. at the out-patient clinic in the hospital, the patient called again and hysterically gave a detailed description of a car accident in which she and her husband were involved. Neither were seriously hurt, but the patient was very upset and emotional. She cancelled her next few appointments because she would be busy taking new roentgenograms and physical exams because of the accident.

About a month later she returned to the physical therapy department and was scheduled to be treated by another therapist, which happens often in the hospital situation. Unfortunately, the patient did not receive a carryover in treatment because of the change in therapists, but remained on program for another few months, and made no substantial improvement.

It is obvious that this patient suffered from intense anxiety, and other manifestations presented under the Preexisting Personality Profile section on page 9. She experienced serious emotional problems, yet continued to defend the position that her somatic pain was the etiology, when, in fact, the opposite was true. Her pain was a defense mechanism for existing, emerging conflicts. She was very reluctant to relinquish it, and when one area responded to treatment, the pain was intense in a new area. This type of patient could spend years in physical therapy, with no substantial relief from physical symptoms. These patients must eventually resolve their conflicts on their own, or receive psychiatric assistance. Otherwise, they will dominate out-patient phsyical therapy departments and be a continuing source of frustration to the therapist unless some insight into their emotional state is realized by both the patient and the therapist.

Depression

Depression may vary from a mild downheartedness or feeling of indifference to a despair beyond hope. In the milder depressive syndrome, the patient is quiet, restrained, inhibited, unhappy, pessimistic, and self-depreciative, and has a feeling of lassitude, inadequacy, discouragement, and hopelessness. The patient is unable to make decisions and experiences difficulty with customarily easy mental activities. He or she is overconcerned with personal problems.

In somewhat deeper depression, there is a constant unpleasant tension; every experience is accompanied by mental pain; the patient is impenetrably absorbed with a few topics of a melancholy nature. Conversation may be painfully difficult. He or she is dejected and hopeless in attitude and manner. The patient's dispirited affective attitude is projected toward his environment, which reflects his or her dolesome outlook. He or she feels rejected and unloved. The patient may be so preoccupied with depressive ruminations that attention, concentration, and memory are impaired.

Depression has its roots in unconscious guilt arising from interpersonal issues, perhaps from unconscious ambivalence and hostility with resentful and aggressive impulses directed toward persons who are the objects of an undesired obligation, or toward persons on whom one is dependent for security. It should be recognized that the effect of depression may include varying degrees of sadness, guilt, and shame simultaneously—sadness because of a loss, guilt over a repressed hostile drive, and shame due to failure to live up to some personal standard (Kolb, 1973).

Depression is so prevalent in low-back patients that it is listed in a separate category as a precipitating factor in Fig. 2a. A psychiatrist at New York Hospital was asked for an estimation of how many of his low-back patients were depressed. He said, "They are all depressed, only the degree changes from patient to patient." Perhaps this is an overestimation, but the point is clear. There is a direct correlation between depression and psychosomatic pain.

Figure 2b shows the cause-and-effect relationship between depression and low-back pain. Depression can help to carry the patient through the gray area between the acute and chronic stages of low-back pain. Because of the pain and accompanying disability of an acute episode, the patient often experiences mild depression. If other precipitating factors are present, or if the depression is severe enough, the patient's pain could continue because of the depression alone, even in the absence of physical pathology. Since 30% (Wilson et al., 1974) of patients experiencing depression manifest symptoms of pain, it is a cycle that is difficult to break without intervention.

Here again, the therapist's role becomes crucial. It is a role encompassing three responsibilities:

1. Proper treatment of the 'acute' episode
2. Proper evaluation following the 'acute' episode
3. Communication with the physician

If any of of these responsibilities are not fulfilled by the therapist, the patient can easily fall into the cycle of the chronically depressed low-back patient.

The Personality Profile of the Low-Back Patient

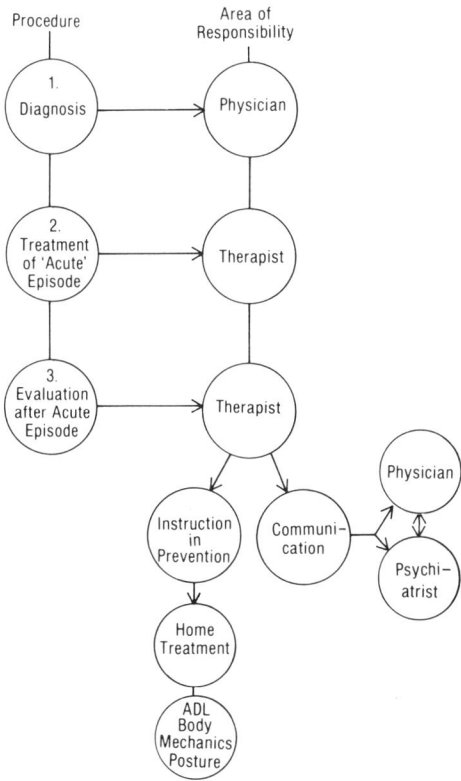

Figure 3.

Figure 3 outlines these areas of responsibility and the options open to the therapist. There are two ways that the therapist can help the patient suffering from an "acute" episode avoid a pattern of chronicity from either depression or other preexisting personality factors. At the proper time during treatment (Fig. 3. No. 3) the therapist and the primary-care physician decide whether or not the sequelae of pain and disability from the initial episode warrant further communication and/or referral to the physician or psychiatrist. If so, the patient is informed, and the proper appointments are made. If the therapist decides that the acute episode has been successfully treated and the patient is ready to return to full function, the patient's treatment time is then extended to include ADL and proper body mechanics. A review of an effective home program, including instructions for relief from muscle spasm, should be reviewed. In this manner, the patient has either (1) an effective treatment for an acute episode, including a preventive home program, or (2) a referral to the proper physician should the acute treatment have failed to return the patient to a relatively pain-free and functional state.

Many times a psychiatrist will prescribe a supportive drug (lithium carbonate and tricyclic antidepressants) for the chronically depressed patient. This can be a successful adjunct to physical therapy. Recently, Kane studied depressed low-back patients who were without x-ray or neurologic finding of disc disease. The patients exhibited clinical symptoms of depression: loss of appetite, sexual interest, and sleep; dizziness; and shortness of breath. He found that treatment with antidepressant drugs proved effective in 80% of the sample, and, in a smaller group where these drugs were compared against physiotherapy, the drugs were found to be far superior.

With some patients, the most effective treatment they can receive will be a referral to the proper physician, and with others it will be a comprehensive exercise program including ADL and body mechanics. Still, there will be other times when listening, caring, and giving emotional support are the only modalities that will help a depressed low-back patient.

Conversion Hysteria

Severe anxiety can be displaced in several different ways; as a phobia, as an anxiety reaction, or, unconsciously, it can be converted into a functional symptom in parts of the body innervated by the sensorimotor nervous system. This "conversion" will lessen the anxiety the patient feels on the conscious level, and usually symbolizes the underlying mental conflict that is productive of the anxiety. "It may for example 'convert' a mental concept into a significant body symptom, as when hysterical paralysis of an arm expresses a wish to do a forbidden act, yet ambivalently prevents its accomplishment (Kolb, 1973). Even though some solution to his or her problem is provided by the resulting symptom, the patient is in no way aware or conscious of the underlying process of a conversion reaction. This is in direct contrast to the *malingerer*, who purposefully and consciously makes up signs and symptoms of mental and/or physical disorders for purposeful gains.

The patient who suffers from a conversion reaction usually has a history of immaturity in the psychosexual and emotional development, and the episode is produced as an escape or relief from some anxiety-producing situation. The patient will experience a "primary gain" in terms of the defense mechanism against the anxiety produced by the symptom. The "secondary gain" is some material or emotional advantage that usually affords a solution to the immediate problem, which is attained by the symptom.

Here are some characteristics of a patient suffering from a conversion reaction (Kolb, 1973):

1. With motor disturbances in hysteria, function is disturbed without demonstrable physiological or anatomical change (i.e., reflexes are usually WNL).
2. The patient presents with a bizarre or unusual account of the symptoms that does not always follow the pattern expected from the described illness.
3. The patient will probably exaggerate minor aches and pains and believe them to be of a disabling degree.
4. Frequently, he appears indifferent and undisturbed by the symptoms (*la belle indifference*).
5. The history often describes the symptoms to be intermittent in nature, and usually exacerbated by incidents of an emotional nature.
6. Should the anxiety-ridden topics or associated subjects be introduced by the therapist, the painful complaints will usually be reiterated and pronounced by the patient.
7. With actual physical disease the patient can tolerate and actually entertains the thought that his pain may be of an emotional origin, but a patient whose pain is psychogenic diligently seeks a physical basis.

Whenever a conversion reaction is suspected, therapists should remember to ask themselves if the patient's signs or symptoms serve some purpose in the patient's life. Although both the malingerer and the patient suffering from a conversion reaction will realize secondary gains, the following differentiations should be noted: the malingerer will often offer statements of discrepancy, contradictions, and an exaggeration of symptoms, whereas the conversion patient will present a more consistent history. The malingerer will usually express much more concern about his symptoms, whereas the conversion patient will display *la belle indifference*.

Although malingering and patients suffering from conversion reactions are much less frequent than depressed, anxiety-ridden patients, it is imperative that the therapist be aware of both categories of patients. These are other instances where even the most exacting physical therapy regime, alone, will not offer relief from pain and/or long-term disability.

Masochism

To patients suffering from severe guilt feelings, pain may actually yield pleasure. Through the growing period children associate punishment with "being bad" and the atonement of guilt. For some children, as well as adults, pain means forgiveness, and finally the acceptance and reunion with loved ones. Pain serves as punishment. Punishment relieves guilt.

"Clinically, we find either a long-term background of guilt and/or an immediate guilt-provoking situation precipitating pain. The clinical characteristics of the chronically guilt-ridden person are not difficult to recognize if one appreciates the role of penitence, atonement, self-denial and self-deprecation as a means of self-inflicted punishment to ease the feeling of guilt. These individuals are chronically depressed, pessimistic and gloomy people whose guilty self-depreciating attitudes are readily apparent from the moment they walk in. They have little joy or enthusiasm for life and some seem to have suffered the most extraordinary number of defeats, humiliations and unpleasant experiences. They seem to drift into situations or submit to relationships in which they are hurt, beaten, defeated and humiliated. When life is treating them the worst, when circumstances are the hardest, their physical health is likely to be at its best and they are free of pain. Paradoxically, when things improve, when success is imminent, a painful symptom may develop. These people do not believe they deserve success or happiness and feel they must pay a price for it. Often these patients seek the infliction of further pain from their physicians, usually in the form of surgery and/or painful diagnostic or therapeutic procedures. Treatment that is not painful or a hardship may be rejected" (Mane, 1977).

Example
> Ms. L. was well known to the physical therapy department. She was a 36-year-old female who spent most of her time as a bed-ridden invalid. She was a known drug-abuser and a difficult patient. This was her sixth hospital admission in a period of four years. She was status post two laminectomies and a cordotomy, and was anxiously awaiting her next surgical procedure, which she referred to often. Her present diagnosis was low-back pain with radiation along the sciatica distribution of the right leg.

During other extended periods of physical therapy Ms. L. had received electric stimulation, massage, heat, cold, exercise, relaxation training, pool therapy, ambulation with various devices, and whatever else was available to her. Each time there was no improvement and she was returned home to resume her role of a bed-ridden nonproductive person.

The present plan was to use the transcutaneous nerve stimulator (TNS) for pain-relief. The appropriate placement of the electrodes and settings were to be taught to the patient so she could continue the treatment at home. She would also receive pool therapy.

The patient arrived on a stretcher because she could not sit for any length of time, nor could she walk because of muscle weakness from disuse atrophy and pain. Ms. L. would not respond to any mode of treatment, nor would she ambulate.

She was unkempt in physical appearance, and was a chain-smoker before, during, and after the treatment. Since nothing else seemed to work, the therapist decided to put the emphasis of the treatment on developing a rapport with the patient.

For the next 3 or 4 days, the therapist showed unusual attention to, and concern for, the patient. At the same time, however, the therapist remained firm and verbally voiced the fact constantly that the patient would obtain enough relief from the TNS unit to be able to walk again. The patient was introduced to other patients and therapists in the department, and she was treated as an acquaintance rather than a patient. She responded well to this treatment.

By the end of the week, the patient suggested, herself, that she try to walk, but only with the assistance of at least two other people. Finally, the patient was transferred from the stretcher, and with maximum assistance she ambulated with a walker the distance of 5 feet. In a period of 2 weeks she was walking 25 feet with visual supervision only. However, whenever the patient felt the therapist was not giving her enough attention, she would stumble and "almost" fall. If she felt she was left in a chair too long, she would "accidentally" push over the walker so someone would call the therapist. The patient was manipulative of the therapist and the environment.

Each time Ms. L. made substantial progress and gained some independence, she would sustain a minor injury that would cause her to regress to the point of dependency. While she was walking in the pool, she "sprained" her ankle, and while ambulating in the department, she "pulled" a hamstring muscle. Each injury was at a time when she was making progress, and just after she was praised consistently by the therapist and others in the department.

Finally, Ms. L. was discharged. Her ambulation status was semi-independent with a walker.

Several months later, Ms. L.'s neurologist contacted the therapist and asked her to see the patient at home. The therapist found Ms. L. in bed, and in the interim since her discharge, she had fallen several times. She had not left her house since returning home, even though she was now ambulating with no device. The patient was put on a mild conditioning program, and was told to leave the house and walk an increasing number of city blocks per day. She was reinstructed in the use of the TNS.

Three weeks later the therapist returned to find the patient on crutches. She once again "sprained" her ankle, this time, in the bathroom. A day or two before that, she fell in the street and cut her hand. She was well known in the emergency room of neighborhood hospitals because of these minor accidents.

In the meantime, Ms. L. continued to self-medicate and was a chronic drug-abuser. At times it was difficult to interpret her speech. She always appeared sleepy, lethargic, and drugged. On several occasions she reported that her TNS unit gave her no relief from pain.

Two weeks later, the patient was readmitted to the hospital for drug abuse. She stayed 10 days and was released. During this period she was uncooperative in physical therapy, which was under the direction of another therapist. She phoned the original therapist and said that she was having personal problems at home. Her drug situation had not changed and she continued to overmedicate herself.

Two weeks later she entered the psychiatric ward of the hospital.

This type of patient can be most frustrating to work with. Just as she reaches a physical plateau, a minor injury occurs, and the patient regresses. The therapist can employ every methodology of treatment available, but the patient progresses only to a semi-independent state, and then goes backwards.

A masochistic type of patient, who needs pain as punishment, is a constant drain on the emotions of the therapist. It is the least rewarding type of low-back patient the therapist can encounter and one that must be pinpointed as early as possible. Effective communication between the therapist, the primary case physician, and the psychiatrist is imperative for the management of this type of low-back patient.

Pain and Loss (Mane, 1977)

The therapist must carefully consider the history of the patient, particularly life events at the time of initial onset of symptoms. Was the patient experiencing real, imaginary, or threatened object loss? This is another precipitant of painful syndromes.

Pain can manifest itself following the death or permanent loss of a loved one, or during the anticipation of such a loss. Stressful life events over which the patient has no control, involving the loss of a loved one, will often cause him to use a party of his own body to symbolize the lost love object. His experiencing pain in this part, assures the continuing presence of the lost person. Unresolved anger toward the lost person usually accounts for the guilt underlying the pain.

Strong Dependency Needs

There is usually a chain-of-events that predisposes the patient to suffer from strong dependency needs. The patient began work at an early age and has spent years at demanding jobs. He is usually a later-born child from a large family, who marries and soon after has children of his own. "Thus, by virtue of providing for others and not being able to fully depend on their own parents as children, he postpones gratification of such needs until a minor injury provided a rational and socially acceptable means of depending on others for emotional and economic support" (Gentry et al., 1972).

The "Need" for Pain

In each of the preceding descriptions of psychosomatic pain there was a "need" for pain. Each patient experienced anxiety or fear, or their derivatives in guilt and shame, which reached intolerable levels of intensity that finally broke through the usual psychological defenses. This was expressed by a painful symptom.

In many cases, the etiology of low-back pain will not be as clearcut, and the therapist must always remember that the presence of a psychosomatic symptom does not exclude concurrent physical pathology, or, vice versa. The search for the etiology of the pain should be an on-going process, with constant reevaluation, *for it is a small percentage of our low-back population that present only with psychosomatic symptoms.*

In most cases the therapist will recognize a conflict within a patient who also exhibits a legitimate rehabilitation challenge. It is only when the symptoms from the psychological conflict interfere with effective treatment of the physical pathology that intervention is necessary.

Example

    Mr. C. was a 50-year-old man who had lived a very active life. He was a former all-star athelete and well known in the small city in which he lived. He was married with four grown children. He worked at the same position for many years, and was successful. He projected an image of being masculine and of having physical and sexual power. His manner was flamboyant and egocentric. He was an avid golfer.

    Mr. C. underwent a discectomy and laminectomy 1 year prior and experienced a resulting osteomyelitis. He remained in a body-cast for four months, and had physical therapy treatments in two hospitals. All rehabilitation efforts failed. The patient became so debilitated and racked with pain that he was forced to crawl on all fours because he could not assume the upright position. With assistance he used a walker to get to and from the car when he had a doctor's appointment.

    Mr. C. had lost all flexibility in the upper and lower back. He had decreased muscle power in the lower extremities and back muscles. Foot drop was present on the right, and he experienced pain with all movements of the back. With forward flexion of the trunk, the patient was 26 inches from the floor. He could perform very few functional activities. He could not bend over enough to drink from a water fountain, and he did not have enough flexibility to put his pants on in the sitting position.

As one would expect, Mr. C. suffered from moderate depression, and was extremely bitter because of his resultant condition. He expressed the desire to sue several of his doctors for malpractice. From the time he arrived as an in-patient Mr. C. announced at least 10 times daily that "he would never be normal again."

Although Mr. C. was cooperative during the evaluation and beginning of his treatment in performing whatever physical movements that were asked of him, he continually verbalized his discontent with all doctors, and the extreme pain he was feeling at the time. He said he knew the treatments "would not work" and that "he would never be normal again." He stopped whoever would listen to him and dominated all conversations with his negativism. He disrupted and disturbed other patients. The therapists who worked with Mr. C. complained that he was abusive, insulting, and difficult to put up with.

Despite Mr. C.'s attitude, intensive physical therapy continued for 3 weeks. His remarks were ignored so that his negative attitudes would not be reinforced with attention, and the patient was continually reminded that every day he was closer to returning "to normal." By the third week the patient could perform all activities including bending, twisting, squatting, and running 10 flights of stairs, he could ride a bicycle and swing a golf club. He could drink from a water fountain, and dress himself. He was only 5 inches from the floor in forward flexion. The only difficulty remaining was in putting shoes and socks on because of a tightness in the internal rotators of the hip. Despite the miraculous progress made by the patient in 3 weeks, he insisted that he was not better and could not perform in activities as he once did.

When the patient complained that he could not perform functional activities, the therapist asked him what he could not do that he wished he could. He replied, "pick up a piece of paper on the floor." The therapist dropped a paper on the floor and asked him to pick it up, which he did. Still, he refused to acknowledge that he could do it. This was repeated with all activities.

Mr. C. left the hospital after 3 weeks of intensive physical therapy. One of his therapist's commented that "Mr. C. got better, in spite of himself."

Two months after his discharge, the therapist did a follow-up home evaluation on Mr. C. He had played nine holes of golf on the preceding two mornings, and had returned to work on a part-time basis. He said that he was still not performing as he did years ago, before his initial episode, and that he doubted he would ever return to that level of participation in his work. His only avid interest at this point was golf. He would be happy, he said, "to quit work altogether, and only play golf nine hours a day." Pain was still Mr. C.'s chief complaint, and he still insisted that "he would never be normal again."

By the end of the second week of his treatment in the hospital, an interview was arranged with his wife, because of Mr. C.'s unusual attitude toward his pain. The therapist explained that for some reason Mr. C. felt that he could not perform in his normal role of husband, father, or provider in the manner in which he had in the past. He used his dependence on the pain to legitimize his lack of performance. In effect the pain syndrome probably arose from a conflict between his desire to be a strong man and perform in his usual manner, and his feelings of weakness and nonproductivity. She was assured, however, that it was possible for Mr. C. to feel some pain in rotational movements because of the nature of his surgery, but certainly not to the degree of dependency that he described. She was asked to allow Mr. C. to perform all functional activities at home on his own, and not let his dependence on pain make him into a physical "cripple" once again. She agreed.

Mrs. C. was also asked about life events surrounding Mr. C.'s prolonged period of disability. She explained that since he had been out of work, new owners had bought and managed Mr. C.'s place of business, and they were not as patient with him as the old proprietors might have been. Mr. C. expected to get fired at any moment. His insecurity in his job, and in his performance in other areas of his personal life, had a major emphasis on his dependence and "need" for pain at this time in his life. It was Mr. C.'s way of coping with an intolerable amount of anxiety arising from internal conflict.

At one point during his hospitalization the patient was seen routinely by a staff psychiatrist. He made no specific recommendations. Mrs. C. was advised by the therapist, however, that if her husband became overly dependent on his pain, and was in danger of becoming a physical "cripple," or, was exposed to any long-term stressful events, it might be advantageous for him to seek further psychiatric help.

Mr. C. is a good example of a patient with a severe emotional conflict who was rehabilitated "in spite of himself" to a functional level of performance. His emotional disability did not block the efforts of the therapist, and he was successfully physically rehabilitated. His "need" for pain, however, was still present after discharge, and he continued to depend on it for emotional stability.

PROGRESSION OF THE LOW-BACK PATIENT

The remainder of Fig. 1 illustrates the possible progression of the low-back patient. Note that 50% proceed to the "chronic" state, which was defined earlier in the text as a time when a patient will experience 3 or more lengthy treatment periods during 1 year, or have his or her functional capabilities decreased substantially over a lengthy period. Certain patients with pain suffer, and certain do not. That is to say that patients who experience the emotion of pain, together with the sensation of pain, are the ones who experience pain and suffering. One theory suggests that we react reflexly to pain with a variety of motor, autonomic, and sensory responses that collectively are considered emotion. This is referred to as the emotion of pain (Wilson et al., 1974). It is merely a description of the patients affective state. It is not surprising, then, that all patients who have both pain and suffering have been found to be depressed and experiencing a state of suffering (Wilson et al., 1974).

On the other hand, patients experiencing pain without suffering, perceive the sensation of pain alone, without the emotion of pain. Their prognosis for recovery from low-back pain is much greater than their counterparts, the patients who experience both pain and suffering.

When a patient who is in a suffering state experiences an acute episode of pain he will usually respond in an emotional manner, in an attempt to get the observer to provide comfort to the individual by relief from the offending stimulus. By and large, this emotional response to pain is culturally determined, and it may be exaggerated by Latins and inhibited by Spartans, Apaches, or Orientals (Wilson et al., 1974). Chronic sufferers respond to long-standing pain with additional emotional components or an intensification of existing ones. A patient can experience both acute and chronic suffering concurrently.

This schematic representation is by no means a one-way street. Suffering patients often return to the "acute" stage where they began the long process that led them into a life of pain and suffering. This returning, "suffering" patient, who is also experiencing an exacerbation of low-back pain, is often the "low-back transient" who presents himself to the therapist as an acute low-back patient.

SUMMARY

The therapist has a choice of one of two roles to assume when treating a low-back patient. He can treat the patient's physical signs and symptoms only, and reduce his services to that of a technician or assistant; or, he can treat the total patient by gaining insight into his personality profile as well as his physical symptoms, and offer a truly professional approach to the relief of low-back pain.

Because the purpose of this chapter is to educate the therapist to the personality processes and their relationship to the patient's propensity to chronicity, the primary emphasis in the theory presented, was one relating to pain of a psychosomatic origin. The therapist's first responsibility, however, is to exhaust all possibilities relating to the treatment of physical symptoms before dismissing the patient as suffering from "emotional" problems. Rather than referring the problem patient to a psychiatrist when an internal conflict is first suspected, the therapist should put the emphasis of the treatment on developing an effective rapport with the patient. Many times a relationship of this type, based on respect and trust, will be the emotional support needed by the patient at a time when he or she is experiencing a stressful life experience, or, an exacerbation, if the patient is an acute sufferer. Only when the emotional manifestation completely interferes with rehabilitation efforts, or the patients ability to cope with the pain or resulting events, should the therapist consider referral to a psychiatrist. At that time psychiatric help should be offered only as an adjunct to physical therapy treatment. The patient must know that he or she is not being deserted by either the primary-care physician or the therapist. Patients should be introduced gently to the idea of seeing a psychiatrist only when they are able to discuss their problems in a meaningful way, and if they are able to relate their pain or other symptoms to a problem they are having. The therapist should never verbalize, or even infer, that the patient's pain "is not real," nor should the therapist promise to cure the pain. The patient should realistically expect some good days and some bad days, regardless of the etiology of pain.

As with other physical therapy situations, the patient should always know the treatment's goal and what is to be accomplished. Whenever possible patients should be kept in an active role, in comparison to the passive role one assumes at the time of surgical intervention or other invasive treatments such as nerve block, etc. This will accomplish two important things for patients; it will force them to assume responsibility for their improvement, and it will afford them some control over their environment. In order that this active role carryover into life situations, it is sometimes necessary to restructure the parts of the patient's life that concentrate on pain or suffering. Occupational therapy can be of benefit here, both in teaching patients new skills, which will add to their independence, and by affording patients the opportunity of group projects and interaction where they can verbalize their feelings in a supportive atmosphere. New social awareness, which is a necessary prerequisite for the patient returning after a prolonged disability, could also be gained in this manner.

Above all, patients must be aware of two components of their therapeutic program at all times. First, they must always know their goal. Each part of the therapy should be explained to the patients. They should know the short-term goal of each exercise. Is it to stretch a muscle, strengthen a postural group, or remove excess tension from a muscle? How does a modality work, and why is it included in the patient's program? In addition, patients should know the long-term goal of their total program, and if there is an emotional component present, how one aspect can interfere with the other. Teaching is one-half of the therapist job, thinking is the other half. Secondly, patients should know, by the therapist's reaction, whether or not they are reaching their goal. For each exercise, as well as their total functional capacity, the therapist should "condition" the positive efforts of patients whenever they perform in the desired manner. When patients reach either short- and/or long-term goals, they should be praised, and rewarded with desirable conversation and attention. With patients who are poorly motivated, the therapist should concentrate on praising the smallest thing that the patient does well, like one simple exercise movement. If coming to the standing position is not possible, instead of emphasizing walking and therefore, defeat, have the patient perform exercise in the chair. Find something the patient does well and reward him or her for it.

This is therapy with a positive effect, and even the most unmotivated patient will respond to it. In order that patients know their goals, and whether or not they are reaching them, the therapist must know at what level the patient is functional, and proceed to set the goals from that perspective.

Successfully treating a low-back patient with pain of an unknown etiology, and/or of a psychosomatic origin, is not impossible. It does, however, demand of therapists all of their professional insight, skills, and dedication.

BIBLIOGRAPHY

Cairns, D. T., Lynn Mooney, V., and Pace, B. J. (1976). A comprehensive treatment approach to chronic low back pain. *Pain 2*(3).
Gentry, D. W., Shows, D., and Thomas, M. (1972). Presented at the 19th Meeting of the Academy of Psychosomatic Medicine.
Kane, F. (1977). Psychological aspects of the pain-prone patient, *Orthop Rev 6*(2).
Kolb, L. (1973). *Modern Clinical Psychiatry.* Saunders, Philadelphia.
Lauder, W. T. (1976). A review of operant conditioning in the treatment of chronic low back pain. *Off J Assoc Rehab Nurses 1*(2).
Nachemson, A. L. (1976). The lumbar spine. An orthopaedic challenge. *Spine 1*(1).
Pheasant, H. C. (1977). Backache—Its nature, incidence and cost. *West J Med 126.*
Raskind, R., and Mead, S. (1967). The low-back derelict. *South Med J.*
Russek, A. S. (1955). Medical and economic factors relative to the compensible back injury. *Arch Phys Med Rehabil 36.*
Sarno, J. E. (1976). Chronic back pain and psychic conflict. *Scand J Rehabil Med 8.*
Schwab, J. J., Fennell, E. B., and Warheit, G., (1973). The epidemiology of psychosomatic disorders. Presented at the Annual Meeting of the Academy of Psychosomatic Medicine.
Tinling, D., and Klein, R. F. (1966). Psychogenic pain and aggression: The syndrome of the solitary hunter. *Psychosom Med 28.*
Westrin, C.-G., Hirsch, C., and Lindegard, B. (1972). The personality of the back patient. *Clin Ortho Related Disroder 87.*
Wilson, W., Blazer, D., and Nashold, B. (1974). Observations on pain and suffering. Read at the Seventh Annual Meeting of the Neuroelectric Society.

Chapter 2

Anatomical Entities Relating to Low-Back Pain

INTRODUCTION

The purpose of this book is to improve the skills of the therapist treating a patient with low-back pain by adding insight into evaluation and treatment concepts and their application. Therefore, a long dissertation on anatomy and basic physiology at this point would be inappropriate. However, Figure 4 is presented to review the interrelationships between the many systems that must coordinate functionally to work in a smooth, efficient manner. When the muscular components and mechanical and psychological stresses are added, it is no wonder that there is no one simple solution to low-back pain and that as many corresponding, and sometimes contradictory, types of treatment are now prevalent. The causes are as different and varied from patient to patient as is each patient's own personality and lifestyle. Until the therapist is able to recognize symptoms relating directly to specific malfunctioning structures, the treatment will not be successful. For the patient's benefit, therefore, it is the responsibility of the therapist to gain a working knowledge of the anatomy of the back, including functional and mechanical considerations.

The following is a glossary-type listing of muscular, structural, discogenic, and neurological considerations that a therapist is most likely to encounter in clinical practice, and are examples of the multifaceted etiologies possible for low-back pain.

MUSCULAR/LIGAMENTOUS CONSIDERATIONS

Increased Muscle Tension

Every muscle has a resting length that it attains when no external forces are acting on it. It is a comfortable and healthy position for

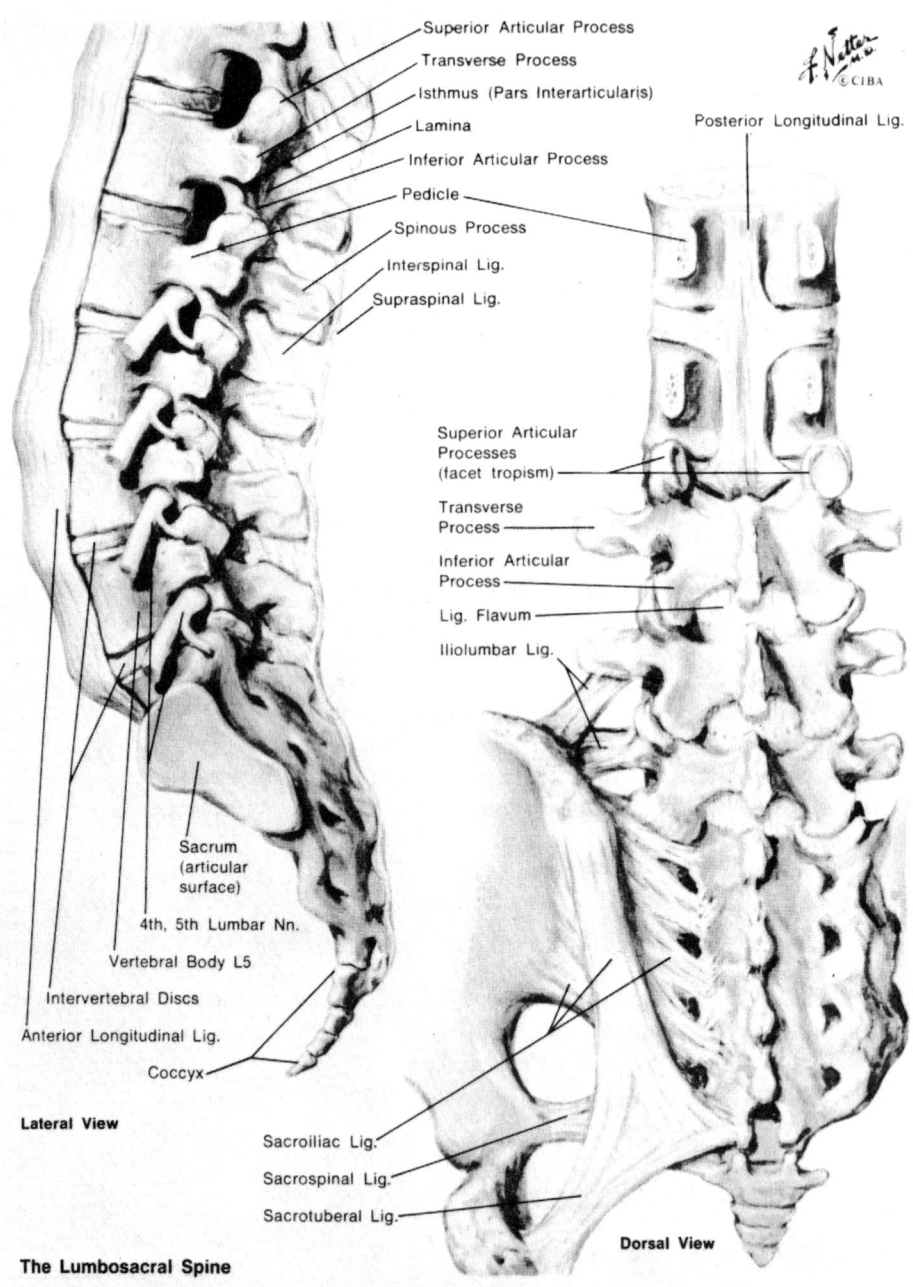

Figure 4.

the muscles to return to after heavy work; however, repeated tensing of a muscle, whether it is caused by internal or external factors, can result in a loss of length and elasticity of that muscle, because it is unable to return to its resting state. Muscle tension alone can be a cause of pain, because painful muscles respond to irritation with increased activity, which in turn, causes more pain.

Muscle Strain

A strain is caused by some form of trauma, usually overstretching and/or overuse. Pain will be elicited from the affected muscle if it is either passively stretched or actively contracted against resistance. Usually, it will be tender to palpation. Active contraction of the muscle should be avoided during the acute state. Ice, compression, and rest are the first considerations.

Ligamentous Sprain

The supraspinous ligament, which extends along the tips of the spinous processes, the articular ligaments around the apophyseal joints, and the anterior and lateral spinal ligaments are most susceptible to sprain. Passive movements that put stress on the involved ligament will cause pain. There will be tenderness along the ligament and at its attachment. Damage to the posterior longitudinal ligament is responsible for some back pain in disc disease, since it is the only part of the surroundings of the disc that contains pain-sensitive endings.

Muscle Inbalance

An inbalance can be caused by muscle weakness or lack of flexibility or both, and must be detected early to prevent further muscular pathology, or more permanent structural deformities (i.e., scoliosis). The weak muscle should be strengthened, the tight one stretched, and the proper emphasis placed on posture.

Muscle Spasm

A spasm is an involuntary contraction of a muscle due to an irritating stimuli. It has been shown that exercise above a minimal level can cause ischemia in the working muscle, and that this lack of local circulation can cause varying levels of pain, probably due to a chemical transfer at the muscle cell membrane, which in turn irritates pain nerve endings. This pain can cause a reflex tonic muscle contraction, which reinforces the ischemic state, and the vicious cycle of muscle spasm is initiated and propagated in this manner. However, overwork is not the only cause of the muscle being in a shortened state and pulled away from its normal resting state. Excessive tension, underwork, fatigue, postural strain, and quick, jerky movements that the body is not prepared for are also causes of muscle spasm.

The most effective treatment for muscle spasm is the immediate application of ice to the entire affected musculature. This slows down considerably the velocity of the pain stimuli input, which allows for a simultaneous return of the muscle to its resting state without reinforcing the cycle of pain, spasm, pain, etc.

The three most common muscles to experience muscle spasm in association with low-back pain are the iliopsoas, hamstring, and paravertebral muscles.

Contusion

The patient experiences a blow to the back, resulting in localized tenderness of the area, and experiences moderate pain on function. In a few hours muscle spasm usually occurs as a protective device to prevent painful motion. Active muscle contraction of the involved muscle is usually not painful, as it is with a muscle strain.

Hematoma Sequelae

Hematoma formation following contusion, gross muscle tearing, or surgery can progress to dense scar formation, which is painful when stretched.

Triggerpoint

A triggerpoint is a local area of tenderness that occurs in a constantly tightened muscle. The blood circulation becomes compromised, which can lead to necrotic muscle fibers. Often these fibers knot up and present as a firm nodule, and in the superficial muscles, are easily palpable. When a muscle is in this tightened state, any sudden or jerky movement can tear muscle fiber, and, again, knot up to form a triggerpoint. Other causes of triggerpoints are exposure to cold, trauma, irritation, emotional tension, muscle spasm, true disc pressure and disc disease, after successful disc surgery or fusion, and with any repeated stressful movements or disturbance of local circulation.

Asymptomatic triggerpoints require no treatment; however, those that do cause pain and limitation of motion require an injection by the physician and follow-up physical therapy as outlined in subsequent chapters.

Piriformis Syndrome

Often times a triggerpoint develops in the piriformis muscle and causes true sciatic radiation, because the sciatic nerve is compromised as it exits the sciatic notch. It is often confused with discogenic pain. The test procedure is included in the following evaluation procedures, and treatment is the same as for other triggerpoints.

Muscle Weakness

Because technology and affluence have afforded most of us a sedentary occupation and lifestyle, muscle weakness has become one of the leading causes of low-back pain. Normally, strong muscles prevent excessive loading on ligaments and joints and offer protection during quick and stressful movements. Muscles of normal strength add the stability and support necessary to prevent injury. Muscles with strength below normal, however, are exposed to possible strain and triggerpoints, and also, provide hazardous conditions for joint vulnerability.

Flexibility

This is a general term for a muscle's ability to stretch to its ultimate length without undue stress or strain to, or resistance from, muscle tissue. Any condition that causes excess tension in the muscle will prevent this natural ability of the muscle.

Contracture

A permanent shortening of a muscle due to the muscle retaining one length for a period of time. It can occur with any pathological shortening of a muscle, spasm, or fibrosis of tissue around a joint.

STRUCTURAL CONSIDERATIONS

Spondylolysis

Specifically, a spondylolysis (Fig. 5) is a bony anomaly of the neural arch causing the posterior unit to split apart, which prevents the

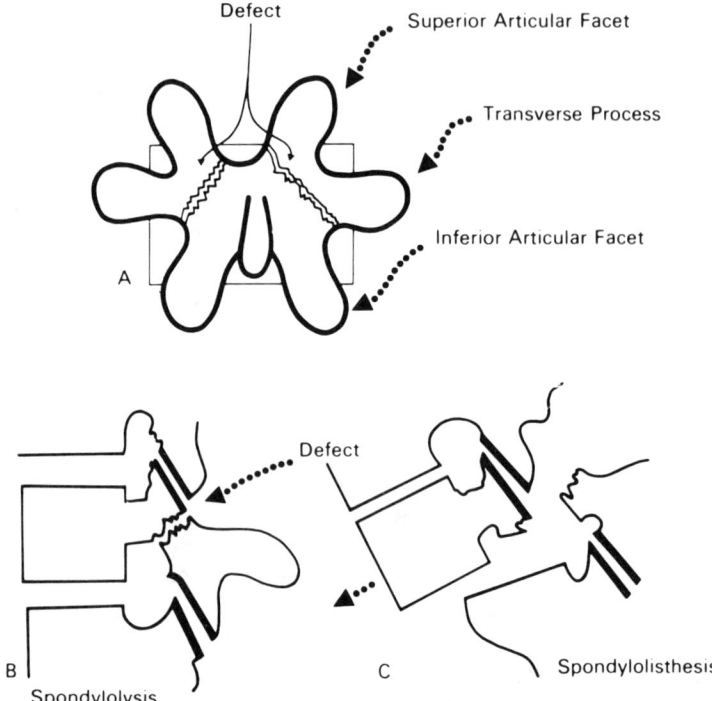

Figure 5. Spondylolytic spondylolisthesis. The basic lesion is a defect in the neural arch across the parts interarticularis (A and B). When degenerative changes occur in the subjacent disc, the vertebral body will displace forward carrying with it the superimposed spinal column and leaving behind the inferior articular facets, the lamina, and the spinous process (C). (Reprited with permission from I. Macnab, *Backache*, Williams & Wilkins, Baltimore, 1977.)

normal gliding movement of the joint. Spondylolysis can be asymptomatic, but it does predispose to premature disc degeneration, which can in itself be painful with local or referred pain in or along the sciatic distribution. Disc degeneration, vertebral instability, and foraminal and extraforaminal encroachment of the nerve root are conditions that frequently are associated with spondylolysis and can be pain-producing.

Spondylolisthesis

This condition can and often does occur as a sequela to the premature degenerative process resulting from spondylolysis. It is a forward subluxation of the body of one vertebra on the vertebra below it (Fig. 5), and occurs most frequently at L_4-L_5 and L_5-S_1. Spondylolisthesis may be asymptomatic; however, the following conditions are examples of what may occur if it progresses: disc rupture at the level above the slip, nerve root compression at the level of the slip, pedicular kinking of the nerve root, or strain of the supraspinous ligament. The patient will usually experience relief from forward flexion or the "stooped" position, and the abnormal wedging of one vertebra on the next will disappear.

Facet Dysfunction

Degenerative changes within the disc, the ligamentum flavum, and the supraspinous ligament cause the zygapophysial (posterior) joints to be vulnerable to strain. These structures usually give stability to the functional unit and allow proper alignment. Normally, the posterior or facet joints guide and direct movement only and are not meant to be weight-bearing joints. However, these degenerative changes cause the joint to be held for prolonged periods at positions that exceed the normal facet alignment, (i.e., in a lordodic position) and cause impingement and irritation of articular synovial tissue.

Since synovial tissue is rich in sensory nerve endings (innervated by the medial branch of the posterior ramus), pain and muscle spasm are a sequalae of this common degenerative process, and normal everyday stress and strain on the back will cause pain. Hyperextension strains should be avoided because they cause a weight shift to the posterior aspect of the vertebral unit.

Scoliosis

Both structural and functional scoliosis disrupt the proper alignment of the posterior facet joints. If the gliding movement of the facet joints are disrupted by such a mechanical influence, the articulating surfaces are no longer working in unison, and friction and impairment occurs. An inflammatory condition of the pain-sensitive synovial lining and articular capsule usually follow.

Muscular considerations of scoliosis also must be considered. A muscle inbalance and other postural considerations are usually present, and make a complete patient assessment a necessity before treatment is instituted.

Osteoporosis

A condition whereby bone reabsorption surpasses bone formation. The exact cause is not known, but many theories have been proposed, including lack of estrogen, long-standing calcium-deficiency, and a high-meat diet that increases hydrogen ion excretion in the urine. The resulting affect is that there is a reduction of total bone mass.

A severe, generalized backache is usually the presenting symptom of osteoporosis, since the vertebral column is mainly affected. The patient usually exhibits a rounded kyphosis in the thoracic region. The trunk is shortened, and the patient has actually lost height. The treatment is concentrated on increasing functional activities and proper therapeutic exercise, together with an increased intake of calcium. The increased activities influences the bodies utilization of the calcium.

Sacroiliac Joint

The pain felt at the sacroiliac joint is usually that of referred pain from the lumbosacral junction due to disc degeneration at that level. Since 75% of trunk flexion occurs at the level of $L_5 S_1$, it is not surprising that this is a common cause of the "ache" in the back.

However, sprains do occur occasionally at the sacroiliac joint, especially below the age of 45, and the presenting symptoms are pain on resistance to hip abduction and weight-bearing, and tenderness at the symphsis pubis. The treatment is usually bedrest, analgesics, bracing, and anti-inflammatory medication.

Osteoarthritis

True osteoarthritis of the spine is a disease of advancing age and trauma. It is a "wear-and-tear" type of arthritis. Degenerative changes can take place both in the body of the vertebra or in the posterior facet joint. As the disc degenerates there is a consequent narrowing of the intervertebral space, and hypertrophy of bone at the joint edges leads to the formation of osteophytes. In the posterior joints there is a wearing away of the articular cartilage and spurring (osteophyte formation). Joint instability occurs with both (see Fig. 6). However, clinically speaking, the instability of the posterior joint is more apt to cause pain and functional interruptions of the unit. This condition can easily lead to a sprain or even subluxation of the facet joint. Treatment usually consists of strengthening supporting structures, correct ADL and body mechanics, and bracing when necessary.

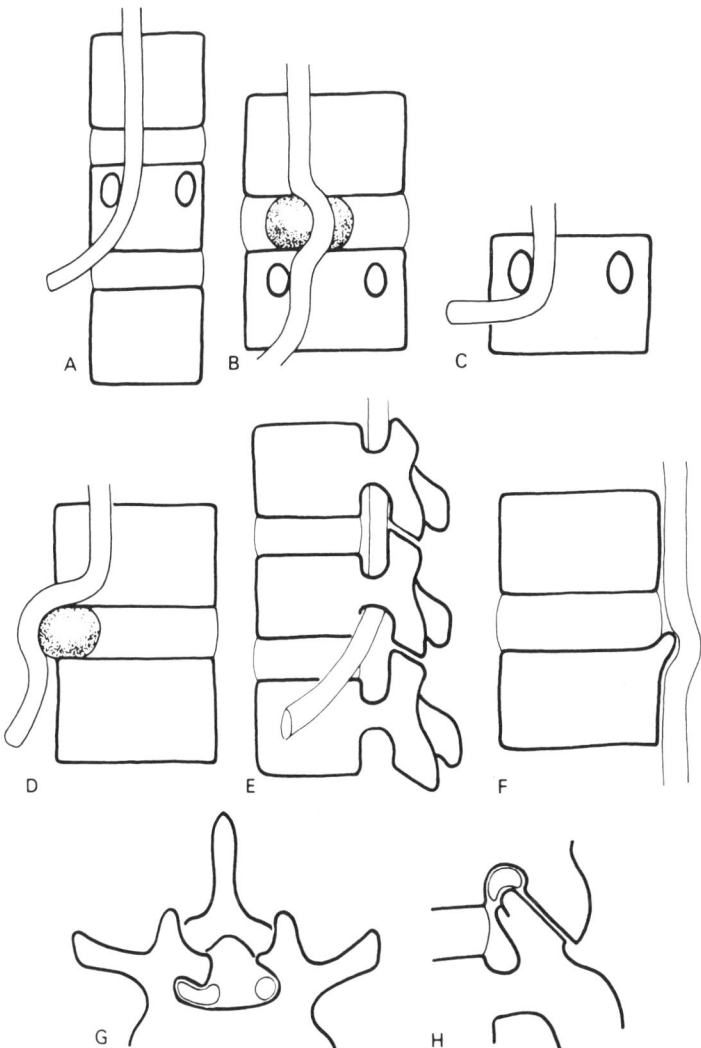

Figure 6. The emerging lumbar nerve roots cross over an intervertebral disc and then sweep around the pedicle before emerging through the intervertebral foramen, at which point they are in contact with the lateral aspect of the disc below (A). It can be seen, therefore, that the nerve root can be compressed by a protrusion of the disc that it passes over (B) by kinking around the pedicle (C), and, after it has emerged through the foramen, by lateral protrusion of the intervertebral disc (D). In the lateral view it can be seen that the nerve root, as it courses down to emerge through the foramen, has to pass underneath the superior articular facet and across the dorsal aspect of the vertebral bodies before it emerges through the foramen (E). The nerve root, therefore, may be compressed by an osteophyte derived from the posterior aspect of a vertebral body (F); it may be compressed as it runs through the subarticular gutter (G); and, finally, it may be compressed in the foramen by the tip of a subluxated superior articular facet (H). (Reprinted by permission from I. Mcnab, *Backache*, Williams & Wilkins, Baltimore, 1977.)

DISCOGENIC/NEUROLOGICAL CONSIDERATIONS (Fig. 6)

Disc Degeneration

Disc degeneration is a normal accompaniment to age and trauma. Part of the gelatinous nucleus pulposus protrudes through a tear in the annulus, usually at the postolateral aspect, its weakest part. Depending on the extent of the herniation, a small bulge will put pressure on the posterior longitudinal ligament and cause pain in the back, whereas a larger herniation will push through the posterior ligament and compress exiting nerve root to cause sciatica. The tear in the annulus is repaired by fibrous tissue, which adds to the loss of normal elastic tissue and functional intactness of the unit. True disc degeneration can lead to segmental instability.

Acute Disc Prolapse

A traumatic insult or a long-standing vertebral instability can be the etiology of an acute disc prolapse. Sciatic scoliosis and/or muscle spasm of the sacrospinalis muscle on the side of the prolapse will be the most evident symptoms. The patient's distress and symptoms will be exaggerated by forward flexion. The treatment is mechanical unloading of the spine, ice therapy, and anti-inflammatory and analgesic drugs until the patient is ambulatory.

Depending on the degree of disc herniation, the resulting disc material will cause pressure on exiting nerve roots, which will cause pain, redness, heat, and swelling in the area of the compromised nerve root. The patient's inactivity will contribute to this build-up of edema that will continue to build and pressure the nerve for at least 72 hours after the initial irritation because of the lack of the "muscle pump" action. This will in turn cause an increase of pain with activity after a period of inactivity, in which time the edema has accumulated. Therefore long periods of complete inactivity should be discouraged, and the patient should be on a program of relaxation and limbering as soon as possible, as discussed in Chap. 5.

Segmental Instability

Hyperextension strains are the most frequent cause of back pain resulting from segmental instability. This disruption in the normal mechanism of the joint causes a constant position of hyperextension at the posterior joint. In this case there is no free-play in the joint; it is held at its physiological limit constantly, so that even a slight day-to-day hyperextension strain will cause irritation and pain. Repeated sprains of the posterior joints will lead to degenerative changes, and true osteoarthritis of the spine as indicated by traction spurs on a roentgenogram. Often, patients will describe this pain as "Lumbago" or "It happens whenever I 'throw my back out'."

Nerve Root Tension

An interruption of the normal exiting of the nerve root by extradural lesion is referred to as nerve root tension. The two most reliable tests to determine this condition is the bowstring sign and limitation of the straight leg raise, both of which are described in detail in Chap. 3.

Nerve Root Irritation

A combination of pressure on the nerve root and an inflammatory response to herniated disc material is referred to as nerve root irritation. It is believed that these combined effects cause peripheral muscle tenderness and a radiation of pain into the hip area, which is often mistaken for hip pathology. The pain of nerve root irritation can be reproduced by the traction placed on the nerve by having the patient assume the "knee-kiss" position.

Nerve Root Pressure

Pressure on a normal nerve does not cause pain, it causes paresthesis. Pressure on a nerve that is already irritated, whether it be from traction on the nerve, by sitting, standing, or any aggravating movement, will cause pain. When the pressure on the nerve has been for a prolonged period, the symptoms will be paralysis, loss of tendon reflexes, and sensory changes.

Herniated Nucleus Pulposus

Synonyms for this term are slipped disc, bulged disc, ballooned disc, prolapsed disc, protruded disc, herniated disc, and ruptured disc. The patient, however, may explain his condition as: "I have a disc" or "I have a pinched nerve."

Other Conditions to be Discounted by the Physician

    Spinal Stenosis

    Viscerogenic Pathology

    Vascular Pathology

Additional Neurogenic Considerations

Ankylosing Spondylitis

Scheuermann's Disease

Rheumatoid Arthritis of Spinal Joints

Intraspinal Lesions

Extraspinal Lesions

SUMMARY

The current literature suggests that the degenerative processess are by far the leading cause of low-back pain. However, muscular etiologies also contribute significantly, and become increasingly evident as the population becomes alarmingly more sedentary. There is no treatment that will counteract normal degeneration, but a strong and flexible supporting structure of healthy muscles can definitely aid in stability and functional capacity of the back.

"Poor body conditioning contributes a significant part to disk degeneration. Insofar as disk nutrition is considered to be by imbibition, the nutrients must be brought to the disk by adequate circulation. The surrounding tissue must be maintained sufficiently flexible to permit tissue-fluid effusion and diffusion. Good muscle tone and contractility are essential in supplying suitable circulation to the region" (Cailliet, 1968).

The therapist should be aware of the multifaceted etiologies of low-back pain together with the interrelationships of the muscular, skeletal, and neurological systems during functional activities. This is a prerequisite to successful assessment of low-back pain.

BIBLIOGRAPHY

Adams, J. (1973). *Outline of Orthopaedics.* Churchill, Livingstone, London.
Cailliet, R. (1968). *Low Back Pain Syndrome.* Davis, Philadelphia.
Ciba Clinical Symposia (1973). Ciba Pharmaceutical Co., Summit, N.J., Vol. 25, No. 3.
Cobb, C. R., DeVries, H. A., Urban, R. T., Leukens, C. A., and Bagg, R. J. (1975). Electrical activity in muscle pain. *Am J Phys Med 54*(2).
Crutchfield, C., and Barnes, M. (1973). *The Neurophysical Basis of Patient Treatment.* Stokesville Publishing Co., Morgantown, W. Va.
DeVries, H. A. (1974). *Physiology of Exercise.* 2nd ed. Wm. C. Brown Co., Dubuque, Iowa.

Distefano, V. (1976). Injuries to the low back and environs. *Athletic Training* *11*(4).
Edgar, M. A., and Ghadially, J. A. (1976). Innervation of the lumbar spine. *Clin Orthop*, Number 115.
Farfan, H. F., Osteria, V., and Lamy, C. (1976). The mechanical etiology of spondylolysis and spondylolisthesis. *Clin Orthop*, Number 115.
Feinstein, B. (1977). Referred pain from paravertebral structures. *Approaches to Validation of Manipulative Therapy*. A. A. Buerger and J. S. Tubis (Eds.). Thomas, Springfield, Ill.
Hood, L. B., and Chrisman, D. (1968). Intermittent pelvic traction in the treatment of the ruptured intervertebral disk, *J Am Phys Therapy Assoc* *48*(1).
Jayson, M. (Ed.) (1976). *The Lumbar Spine and Back Pain*. Sector Publishing Ltd., London.
Knight, K. (1976). The effects of hypothermia on inflammation and swelling. *Athletic Training* *11*(1).
Kraus, H. (1970). *Clinical Treatment of Back and Neck Pain*. McGraw-Hill, New York.
Lowdon, B. J., and Moore, R. J. (1975). Determinant and nature of intramuscular temperature changes during cold therapy. *Am J Phys Med* *54*(5).
Mcnab, I. (1977). *Backache*. Williams & Wilkins, Baltimore.
Magora, A. (1976). Conservative treatment in spondylolisthesis. *Clin Orthop*, Number 115.
Manual of Orthopaedic Surgery (1972). Published by the American Orthopaedic Association.
Mennell, J., and Zohn, D. (1976). *Musculoskeletal Pain*. Little, Brown, and Co., Boston.
Mooney, J., and Robertson, J. (1976). The facet syndrome. *Clin Orthop*, Number 115.
O'Donoghue, D. (1970), *Treatment of Injuries to Athletes*. Saunders, Philadelphia.
Paine, K. W. E. (1976). Features of lumbar spinal stenosis. *Clin Orthop*, Number 115.
Rosenberg, N. J. (1976). Degenerative spondylolisthesis. *Clin Orthop*, Number 115.
Troup, J. D. G. (1976). Mechanical factors in spondylolisthesis and spondylolysis. *Clin Orthop*, Number 117.
Urbaniak, J. (1976). Basic anatomy and biomechanics of the low back in relation to low back pain. *Athletic Training* *11*(3).

Chapter 3

Evaluation MD/PT

INTRODUCTION

A complete assessment of the patient's status is a necessity before any treatment modality is initiated. The only exception to this is when the patient presents with painful muscle spasm, in which case the physician will give a preliminary examination and take a complete history. The therapist will proceed with treatment of the spasm (as detailed in Chap. 5), both to relieve pain and to expose underlying causes of the pain and spasm. When the symptoms have subsided substantially, either the therapist or the physician will carry out the following skeletal, muscular, neurological, functional, and pain assessments. The assessments will then be analyzed by the physician and the therapist, and jointly, an appropriate treatment regimen will be written specifically for the individual patient. Only in this manner can a successful solution be offered to the patient suffering from low-back pain.

ASSESSMENT FORMS

The following pages are designed as a worksheet for the therapist. They contain all of the pertinent information in an organized manner so that the next step of analyzing the assessments can be accomplished in the most efficient and competent way. The information is arranged by systems, so that it might be established, for example, that the patient's main etiology of pain is in the skeletal system, but that symptoms are also present in the muscular system. In some cases, it is these symptoms that will be the basis for our treatment. Therefore, it is important to differentiate between pain from a structural, muscular, and functional etiology. These worksheets are designed to assist the therapist in accomplishing this differentiation.

If time is at a premium, the assessments can be performed during the first two visits to the therapist (unless an acute muscle spasm is present). However, since the therapist becomes familiar with the tests and the arrangement of the worksheet, the complete assessment should not take more than 1 hour. In addition, if the therapist is operating in a hospital setting, much of the information will be established by the consulting physician and by the chart. When this is the case, the therapist can perform whatever test where results are not available, and reevaluate the other information at a convenient time.

Each assessment has a column marked WNL (within normal limits) for the therapist's convenience. This column can be checked whenever there is nothing significant to be noted. The muscle tests require only a circling of the proper grade, and the functional assessments need just a quick check mark. The same worksheet can be used for a long period of time, by using a different color of pen for each evaluation. For example, a blue pen can be used the first time, a red pen the second time, and a black pen for the third reevaluation. Consideration should always be given to the most efficient use of both the patient's and the therapist's time and energy expenditure.

Name _____   Age _____
History # _____   Dx _____
Date _____   Examiner _____

Skeletal Assessment

Chest measurement   at rest _____ in.
(over xyphoid bone)   maximum inspiration _____ in.
                         maximum expiration _____ in.

Shoulder height
                    right to left WNL _____ or _____
Inferior angle of scapula from spine   R _____ in.   L. _____ in.

Observe:	WNL	
Cervical Lordosis	_____ or	_____
Dorsal Kyphosis	_____ or	_____
Lumbar Lordosis	_____ or	_____
Level of iliac crests	_____ or	_____
Leg Length (standing position)	_____ or	_____
(supine measurement)	_____ or	_____
Medial Arches	_____ or	_____
Sacro Iliac Compression	_____ or	_____
Bilateral SLR	_____ or	_____
Spondylolisthesis	_____ or	_____

(wedging at L/S angle)

Scoliosis (draw the curve)   Structural _____   Functional _____

Spinous Processes, rotated, immobile, etc.
  (forward flexed position)   _____ or _____ At: _____
  (supine position)   _____ or _____ At: _____

Other Abnormalities:

X-Ray Findings:

Name _____ Age _____
History # _____ Dx _____
Date _____ Examiner _____

Muscular Assessment (1)

Palpation

Muscle Tenderness	WNL	PRESENT
Calf (S_1)	_____ or	_____
Anterior Tibialis (L_5)	_____ or	_____
Quadriceps (L_4)	_____ or	_____

Spasm	WNL	PRESENT
Upper Back	_____ or	_____
Paravertebral Muscles	_____ or	_____
Gluteal	_____ or	_____
Tensor Fasca Lata	_____ or	_____
Hamstring	_____ or	_____
Hip Flexor	_____ or	_____

Fibrositis	WNL	PRESENT
Upper Back	_____ or	_____
Paravertebral Muscles	_____ or	_____
Upper Arms	_____ or	_____
Ankle	_____ or	_____
Sole of Foot	_____ or	_____

Triggerpoints	WNL	PRESENT
At Each Spinous Process	_____ or	_____
Sacroiliac Joints	_____ or	_____
Iliac Crests	_____ or	_____
Greater Trochanters	_____ or	_____
Upper Back	_____ or	_____
Paravertebral Muscles	_____ or	_____
Gluteal	_____ or	_____
Tensor Fasca Lata	_____ or	_____
Hamstrings	_____ or	_____
Calf	_____ or	_____
Other Areas of Pain	_____ or	_____

Name _____ Age _____
History # _____ Dx _____
Date _____ Examiner _____

Muscular Assessment (2)

Functional Muscle Test (Kraus-Weber Test)*

Abdominals	1 2 3 4 5 6 7 8 9 10
Hip flexors	1 2 3 4 5 6 7 8 9 10
Abdominals and Hip flexors	1 2 3 4 5 6 7 8 9 10
Upper Back Extensors	1 2 3 4 5 6 7 8 9 10
Low Back Extensors	1 2 3 4 5 6 7 8 9 10

Specific Muscle Test

Circle
First Test in Blue on _____
Re-evaluation in Red _____

	RIGHT	LEFT
Hip Flexion (L_2)	O T P F G N	O T P F G N
Hip Abduction ($L_{2,3,4}$)	O T P F G N	O T P F G N
Hip Abduction ($L_{4,5}, S_1$)	O T P F G N	O T P F G N
Knee Extension (L_4)	O T P F G N	O T P F G N
Big Toe Extension (L_5)	O T P F G N	O T P F G N
Ankle Dorsiflexion ($L_{4,5}$) Heel Walking	O T P F G N	O T P F G N
Ankle Plantarflexion (S_1) Toe Raises	O T P F G N	O T P F G N

*Figure drawings taken from *Clinical Treatment of Back and Neck Pain* by H. Kraus. Copyright © 1970 by McGraw-Hill, Inc. Used with permission of McGraw-Hill Book Company.

Name	Age
History #	Dx
Date	Examiner

Muscular Assessment (3)

Flexibility		WNL		CIRCLE
Hamstring	R	____	or	∡
	L	____	or	∡
Hip Flexor	R	____	or	Limited
	L	____	or	Limited
Tensor Fasca Lata	R	____	or	Limited
	L	____	or	Limited
Gastrocnemius Soleus	R	____	or	Limited
	L	____	or	Limited
Rectus Femoris	R	____	or	Limited
	L	____	or	Limited
Lower Back/Hamstrings eliminated (forward flexion sitting)		____	or	Limited
Lower Back and Hamstrings (forward flexion standing)		____	or	Inches from floor

Muscle Atrophy

Paraspinal	____ or ____
Gluteals	____ or ____
Upper Back	____ or ____
Quadriceps	____ or ____
Calfs	____ or ____
Toe Extensors	____ or ____

Name _____ Age _____
History # _____ Dx _____
Date _____ Examiner _____

Neurological Assessment

Reflexes

Knee Jerk (L_4 Spinal Nerve Reflex Arc)   WNL ____ or ($\downarrow\uparrow$) _____ R or L
Andle Jerk (S_1 Spinal Nerve Reflex Arc)   WNL ____ or ($\downarrow\uparrow$) _____ R or L

Sensation

Check for *pinprick* over portions of leg, compare bilaterally:

    Anterior Thigh   R to L   WNL ____ or _____
    Lateral Thigh   R to L   WNL ____ or _____
    Medial Thigh   R to L   WNL ____ or _____

Check for *numbness*, *tingling*, and the feeling of something *"running"* down the leg:

    L_4 Anteromedial aspect of thigh and knee _____
    L_5 Lateral leg, and the web of the great toe _____
    S_1 Back of calf, lateral heel, foot, and toe _____

Straight Leg Raising

Passive SLR	R WNL ____ or _____	L WNL ____ or _____
La Seque SLR	R WNL ____ or _____	L WNL ____ or _____
Sitting SLR	R WNL ____ or _____	L WNL ____ or _____
Crossover SLR	R WNL ____ or _____	L WNL ____ or _____
Bowstring	R WNL ____ or _____	L WNL ____ or _____

Additional Tests

Femoral Stretch	R WNL ____ or _____	L WNL ____ or _____
Ely's Test	R WNL ____ or _____	L WNL ____ or _____

Inspection

Psoriatic Lesions	yes _____	no _____	where _____
Cafe Au Lait Spots	yes _____	no _____	where _____
Tufts of Hair	yes _____	no _____	where _____
Gluteal Crease R to L (even?)	yes _____	no _____	
Other	_____		

Name _____ Age _____
History # _____ Dx _____
Date _____ Examiner _____

Functional Assessment

Can the patient freely and correctly, using proper Body Mechanics:

Roll from side to side	yes _____	no _____
Come to a side sitting position	yes _____	no _____
Roll up to a sitting position	yes _____	no _____
Sit in a long-sitting position	yes _____	no _____
Come from sitting to standing position	yes _____	no _____
Bend properly to pick up an object on the floor	yes _____	no _____
Lift the object	yes _____	no _____
Carry an object	yes _____	no _____
Walk with a normal gait	yes _____	no _____
Run up a flight of stairs	yes _____	no _____
Sit properly	yes _____	no _____
Lie properly	yes _____	no _____
Sleep properly	yes _____	no _____

Check

Lumbar Pelvic Rhythm during forward flexion	WNL _____	or _____
Extension, returning to the upright	WNL _____	or _____
Side Bend	WNL _____	or _____
Rotation	WNL _____	or _____
Supine, forehead to knee position	WNL _____	or _____
Hip ROM (pain?)	WNL _____	or _____

Name _____ Age _____
History # _____ Dx _____
Date _____ Examiner _____

Pain Assessment (1)

When did it start?

Was it associated with injury?

What other treatment have you had?

When is it aggravated?

by rest	yes _____ no _____
during the night	yes _____ no _____
by sitting	yes _____ no _____
coming to standing	yes _____ no _____
by movement only	yes _____ no _____
by walking	yes _____ no _____
on changing positions	yes _____ no _____
by coughing/sneezing	yes _____ no _____
other	_____

What kind of pain?

Stiffness in the morning	yes _____ no _____
Does it disappear with rest	yes _____ no _____
Is it unremitting regardless of position	yes _____ no _____
Is it continuous	yes _____ no _____
Is it intermittent	yes _____ no _____
Is there numbness or tingling	yes _____ no _____

Which activities have been excluded by the patient because of pain?

Any bowel or bladder problems?   yes _____ no _____

Name _____ Age _____
History no. _____ Dx _____
Date _____ Examiner _____

Pain Assesment (2)

Where is the Pain ?

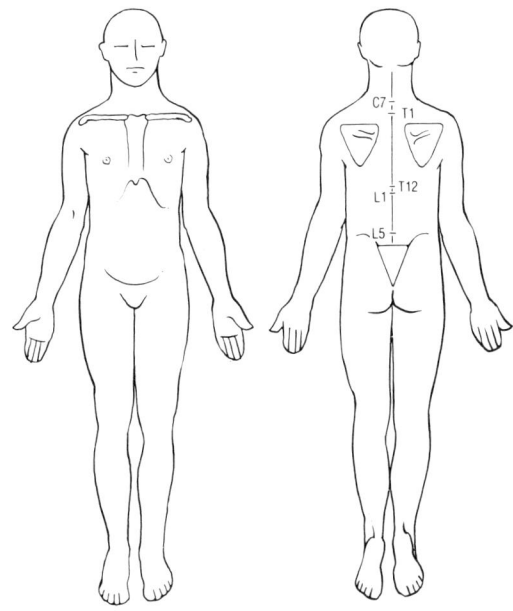

Shade in painful area:
- ↻ ↺ rotation R or L
- = spasm
- ⋁ stiff segment
- ⊗ triggerpoint
- ⧚ fibrositis

EXPLANATION OF MEASUREMENTS

Chest Measurement: Ankylosing spondylitis usually affects men in their second or third decade of life. It begins as a lesion of the sacroiliac joints that usually progresses upward in the spine. The first noticeable change will be a fuzziness or unclear view of the sacroiliac joint on a roentgenogram. A squareness of the vertebral bodies is also characteristic. In addition, pulmonary fibrosis is also a common feature, which leads to a decrease in the movement of the rib cage. This results in loss of pulmonary function, and a decrease of chest expansion is often a leading clinical diagnostic sign. A wasting of the paraspinal muscles will be evident in chronic cases. The patient will also complain of morning stiffness, which is characteristic of an inflammatory reaction. The therapist will note by observation and palpation that the spinous processes do not separate normally during forward flexion. Consequently, there will be a loss of flexion and in some cases, the patient will lose the ability to reverse the lumbar lordosis.

Observation of the *height of the shoulders* and the measurement of *distance of the inferior angle of the scapulae from the spine* give an overall posture. Abnormalities can indicate the presence of scoliosis, muscle weakness, structural deformity, etc.

The *cervical lordosis* and *dorsal kyphosis* are inspected by observation.

The *lumbar lordosis* is measured with a goniometer. One arm is placed vertically against the sacrum, the other is held perpendicular to the floor: 160 to 165 is a normal range. An increase in the lumbosacral angle increases the amount of shearing stress at the lumbosacral joint, and forces the facet joint to become weight-bearing because of a decrease in the posterior disc space. This can cause an irritation and impingement of the synovial lining, which can be pain-producing.

Level of the iliac crests can be observed by having the examiner stand in front of the patient, and place the fingertips of one hand on each crest. The level of the iliac crests should correspond to approximately that of the fourth lumbar vertebra. An inequality in height of the hands is easy to recognize.

Equal leg length is best confirmed by a level pelvis and a straight spine. When a leg length discrepancy is present its influence on the pelvis will usually be evident. If this is the case, lifts in increments of

1/8 inch thickness can be placed under the shorter leg until the pelvis is equal. In the supine position, a tape measure can be used to measure between the anterior superior iliac spine to the medial malleolus to confirm any discrepancy found on observation. In the long-sitting position any differences between the same two points may be due to rotational problems at the pelvis, especially if there is no difference in leg length in the supine position.

The *medial arches* should be checked for depression or flattening. The patient with flat feet should consider arch supports or a visit to the podiatrist, as fallen arches can cause an unequal weight distribution throughout the lower extremities, and, eventually, back pain.

Sacroiliac Compression: Patients over age 45 rarely experience true sacroiliac sprains because the anterior capsule of the sacroiliac joint is ossified by this age. If the patient does feel pain in this area, it is usually referred pain from the lumbosacral area due to disc degeneration. However, two additional tests for sacroiliac sprains are: Have the patient lie on the side, and apply compression downward to the pelvis. This will stress the sacroiliac joints. Secondly, the therapist can resist hip abduction on the side that the patient experiences pain. If pain is experienced over the sacroiliac joint, there is a possibility of a joint lesion.

Active *bilateral straight leg raise* causes hyperextension of the lumbar spine or increased lumbar lordosis. In the presence of disc disease with resulting vertebral instability, this movement will cause pain in the lumbar area.

Spondylolisthesis is usually apparent by the wedging effect visible at the lumbosacral junction on a roentgenogram.

Scoliosis present usually as a functional "C" thoracic curve to the left, or an "S" curve, with the primary curve in the thoracic area being to the right, accompanied by a left lumbar compensatory curve. A left "C" thoracic curve will be accompanied by vertebral rotation to the left, a high left shoulder, scapular abduction, and the ribs will be pulled backward to the left. If the curve is functional, it will disappear on forward flexion. If not, structural changes have already taken place. Having the patient bend sideways is another test of rigidity of the curves. Using an "S" curve as an example, the patient will bend toward the right, which is in the direction of the convexity of a right thoracic curve. If this curve remains and the lower lumbar curve to the left disappears when the patient leans to the left, then the thoracic curve is termed the primary curve and the lumbar is termed the compensatory curve. It is evident that greater structural changes have taken place in the primary curve.

Spinous processes should be examined in both the forward flexed position and with the patient prone. In the forward flexed position the therapist should check by palpation for mobility between each succeeding spinous process, and their alignment in relation to the preceding one. Is one vertebra rotated? Is it fixed in relation to the movement of the rest of the spine? Does the same amount of movement take place at each segment? In the prone position, the therapist should palpate each spinous process. If a tender spot is located, put moderate pressure on the spinous process by pushing in a forward and rotary direction. This is a clinical reproduction of pain resulting from vertebral instability.

MUSCULAR ASSESSMENT (1)

Muscle Tenderness

Muscle tenderness is commonly associated with nerve root irritation. With irritation of S_1 nerve root, the calf becomes tender; with irritation of the L_5 nerve root, the anterior tibialis is tender; and with irritation of L_4, the quadriceps are tender.

Spasm

Spasm is a continuous painful contraction of a muscle over a prolonged period. Either a part of a muscle or the entire belly may be involved. The muscle is hard and shortened, and movement is limited and painful.

Fibrositis

Fibrositis is an unclear entity. It is discounted by some, and defined by others. However, there is no doubt, clinically, that there is such a condition consisting of an inflammation of the muscle and subcutaneous tissue, with pain and a limitation of movement ensuing. The skin should be picked up, or pinched by the therapist, and rolled between the fingers. Any painful resistance to this rolling can be termed fibrositis and should be treated with heat, kneading massage, and active motion of involved parts.

Triggerpoints

Triggerpoints can be palpated by the therapist as small hard nodules. The fingertips should be used to examine all muscles listed and any other painful areas. Bothersome triggerpoints will cause the patient to express pain both verbally and facially, and only those that cause pain should be treated. A triggerpoint is usually not palpable when the muscle is in spasm.

MUSCULAR ASSESSMENT (2)

Functional Muscle Test (Kraus-Weber Test)

This is a gross test of the postural muscles. A grade of 10 denotes the minimum amount of strength necessary to perform activities without strain. Any grade below 10 is an indication for strengthening exercises.

Abdominals

Have the patient lie supine, hands behind neck with knees bent and heels close to the buttocks. The therapist will hold down the heels and request the patient to tuck the chin and roll up to a sitting position. If the patient can roll all the way up, he receives a grade of 10; one-half way up is a grade of 5. The other numbers are used for subjective grades in between these two divisions.

Hip Flexors

Have the patient lie supine, and with both legs extended request the patient to raise both legs up until they touch your hand, and hold this position. The therapist will hold his or her hand about 10 to 12 inches above the plinthe, and will slowly count to ten. If the patient holds the position without strain for the 10 seconds, a grade of 10 is given, for 5 seconds, a grade of five, etc. Pain and straining should be noted.

Abdominals and Hip Flexors

Have the patient lie supine with legs extended, hands behind the neck. The therapist will secure the patient's ankles, and request the patient to tuck the chin and roll up to a sitting position. The same system of grading that is used for the "Abdominal" test is used here.

Upper Back Extensors

Have the patient lie prone with two pillows under the abdomen; hands are behind the neck. The therapist secures the patient's ankles, and requests the patient to raise his or her chest up off the table and hold this position. Make sure the patient's back does not arch. The therapist will slowly count to 10. The patient receives a grade comparable to the amount of seconds the position can be held. Pain and straining should be noted.

Low Back Extensors

Have the patient lie prone, with two pillows under the abdomen; the hands will be put in any comfortable position. The therapist will secure the patient's upper back and request that both legs be kept straight and raised off the table. The grading is the same as for upper back extensors.

Specific Muscle Test

Thse muscle tests are done in the usual manner, as described in the Muscle Testing Manual.

MUSCULAR ASSESSMENT (3)

Flexibility

The maximum length a muscle can attain *actively*.

Hamstrings

Patient lies supine with one leg extended. The other leg is raised straight up in the air as far as possible without straining. Special care must be taken to keep the knee straight throughout the test. Measure by the angle at the hip. Normal is 75 to 90. Repeat other side.

Hip Flexor

Patient will lie supine with both knees bent, feet flat on the table. The patient will raise one knee up to the chest and hold it there tightly with the hands. The patient will extend the other leg out straight and push the back of the knee of this leg into the mat. If lack of flexibility is present, a pull will be felt in the top of the hip area of the extended leg. Repeat on other side.

Tensor Fascia Lata

Patient is sidelying with bottom leg held in 90° of flexion at the hip. Stabilize the pelvis with one hand and with the other lift the top leg upward and back. The pelvis should not rotate. Let go of the leg and gently push downward above the knee to feel the resistance of the lateral thigh structure. If the thigh remains high off the table, tightness is present.

Gastrocnemius Soleus

Patient will stand an arm's length away from a wall. With palms on the wall, heels on the floor throughout the exercise, and the body kept straight, the patient bends elbows and rests against wall with forearms. Check to see if heels are still on the floor, and buttocks should be tucked under. If lack of flexibility is present in the gastrocnemius, it will be felt in this position. The patient remains in this position, and slightly bends the knees. If tightness is felt in this position, it is the soleus that has a lack of flexibility. (An added stretch will be put on each muscle if the test is done on one leg at a time.)

Rectus Femoris

The patient will lie at the edge of the table so that the left leg will be extended off the table. The patient will hold the left ankle and flex the knee as much as possible. The therapist should put slight pressure on the thigh, pushing downward. If tightness is present, the patient will feel a pull in the anterior thigh structure at the hip.

Lower Back/Hamstrings Eliminated

The patient will sit in a straight back chair, with feet on the floor and hands between knees. The patient will tuck the chin and slowly roll down as far as possible. There should be no straining or bouncing. The normal position, which denotes no lack of flexibility, is when patient's chest can reach a parallel position with his thighs.

Lower Back and Hamstrings

The patient will stand with feet shoulder width apart, and hands relaxed at the side. The patient will tuck the chin and slowly roll down as far as possible without strain or bouncing. The knees will be kept straight throughout the exercise. The distance between the fingertips and the floor will be measured in inches.

MUSCLE ATROPHY

The muscle groups listed on the evaluation sheet will be checked for atrophy either by circumference measurement (calfs, quads, etc.) or by visual inspection (paraspinal gluteals, etc.). Points of reference used in measurements should be listed.

NEUROLOGICAL ASSESSMENT

Reflexes

A diminished knee jerk is indicative of an L_4 lesion, whereas a diminished ankle jerk may indicate a S_1 lesion. However, it is important to realize that a diminished reflex activity may result from previous episodes of nerve root compression. This clinical sign of a diminished reflex should be used in conjunction with other diagnostic test results to confirm disc herniation and nerve root compression.

Pin Prick Bilaterally

The therapist will start at the medial aspect of the thigh, and scratch lightly down along the inner leg, medial malleolus, out to the big toes. This will be repeated, starting at the anterior thigh, knee, big toe, and lateral thigh, until the lateral aspect of the foot and toe is included. The patient should compare subjectively the sensation of one leg to the other, and be aware of any difference.

Sensation

The patient will experience numbness, tingling, or the sensation of something "running" down the leg, as listed on the worksheet.

Passive Straight Leg Raise (SLR)

The patient will lie supine with both legs extended. The therapist will raise one leg as high as possible without causing pain, while supporting under the heel and knee. This test must be done slowly and carefully. If the patient feels pain along the sciatic nerve between the ranges of 30° to 70°, it can be indicative, but not conclusive, that a lower segment of the spine is involved. This is in contrast to the patient whose sciatic pain is reproduced by forward flexion of the trunk, and indicates that the involved segment is one of a high level, L_3, L_4, for example, rather than at the lumbosacral junction, or S_1.

LaSeque Sign

The LeSeque sign is performed at the conclusion of the above straight leg raise. When the patient reaches the point of pain, the therapist will lower the leg a few degrees, and dorseflex the ankle. This puts further stretch on the sciatic nerve. The therapist should remember that inflexible hamstring or spasm of the hamstrings can also be confused with a positive SLR.

Sitting Straight Leg Raise

The sitting straight leg raise is performed when the patient is sitting in a chair, and is a good test for either detecting malingering or substantiating a positive SLR. The therapist will extend the patient's knee while examining the ankle, as a disguise, to a level that would be equal to a 90° SLR. If the patient had a positive SLR and no reaction in the sitting position, it would be cause for further investigation. However, the positive SLR may be substantiated if the patient expresses pain either by facial expression or by leaning backward to reduce the stretch on the sciatic nerve, as the therapist extends the knee.

Crossover Straight Leg Raise

The crossover SLR is merely a straight leg raise performed on the unaffected side which reproduces sciatic pain on the affected side. This is usually a conclusive sign of nerve root compression.

Bowstring Test

The bowstring test is a variation of the SLR and is the most conclusive of all SLRs. The therapist raises the patient's affected extremity to a height where pain is reproduced, and then lowers it a few degrees and allows the knee to bend slightly. The patient's foot will be brought to rest on the therapist's shoulder. The actual test is one of applying firm pressure with the thumbs to the popiteal nerve. The patient should be advised in advance of this pressure, so as to avoid any sudden, unexpected movements that might increase the pain. The three most important tests to determine root tension caused by a herniated intervertebral disc are a positive SLR, further aggravated by dorsiflexion (LaSeque sign), and a positive bowstring sign.

ADDITIONAL TESTS

Femoral Stretch

When the patient experiences pain along the anterior aspect of the thigh there is a possibility of compression of the L_4 nerve root. Have the patient lie prone. The therapist will hold at the patient's knee level and hyperextend the hip, while allowing slight flexion of the knee. Some pain may be experienced in the low-back area because of the increased lordosis caused by the hyperextension of the back; however, the test is positive only if the radiating pain is reproduced along the front of the thigh.

Ely's Test

Ely's test gives a good indication of the flexibility of the rectus femoris. The patient lies prone. Passively, the therapist flexes the knee fully. If there is any shortening of the muscle, the patient's hip will flex and rise slightly off the table. In patient's who are experiencing L_4 nerve root irritation, pain in the quadriceps will also be present.

INSPECTION

Psoriatic lesions

Patients with psoriatic lesions have an increased incidence of suffering from either psoriatic sacroilitis or spondylitis. The therapist must keep in mind, however, that additional mechanical factors can also be a contributing factor, even though definite systemic manifestations are present.

Cafe au lait spots, tufts of hair, and other changes in the skin including neurofibromas, polyps, and port wine or anemic nevi often indicate the presence of neurofibromatosis. Tufts of hair can indicate a pilonidal cyst or spina bifida occulta.

Gluteal crease may be uneven, owing to the fact that the gluteus maximus is supplied by the S_1 nerve root. Lesions of S_1 may cause weakness, unilaterally, resulting in uneven gluteal creases.

FUNCTIONAL ASSESSMENT

The functional assessments are self-explanatory. The patient should not be asked to perform movements which cause excruciating pain, and if that is the case, then this part of the evaluation should be postponed. However, if the patient is able, this assessment of functional activities will assist the therapist in setting long-term goals and will also be used as a means of patient-motivation, as will be explained in Chap. 5.

ADDITIONAL MOVEMENTS TO CHECK

Lumbar Pelvic Rhythm

Lumbar pelvic rhythm during forward flexion should be observed closely since it can furnish additional clues to the patient's condition. Failure of the lumbar lordosis to reverse can mean pathology in muscles, joints, ligaments, or capsules. Muscle spasm may be preventing normal movement. It could also indicate hip pathology, tight hamstrings, or an irritated sciatic nerve. This is also a good opportunity to examine the spinous processes for hyper- and hypomobility.

Extension

Extension, returning to the upright position from forward flexion, can put strain on the posterior facets and, together with protective muscular contraction, will compress the facets even further, and cause them to become weight-bearing. Pain will also be elicited if the patient assumes his lumbar lordosis before the pelvis can return to its normal position. This action is characteristic of patients with disc degeneration, as it relieves the strain on the posterior joints as the patient assumes the upright position. This motion of assuming the lumbar lordosis and correct return of the pelvis is normally achieved simultaneously.

Side Bend

Lateral flexion is measured by how far the patient can slide his hand down along the lateral aspect of the thigh toward his knee.

Rotation

The patient is asked to put his hands on hips and turn as far as possible without strain to one side, and then the other. The therapist visually compares one side to the other, and establishes whether or not pain is elicited.

Supine, Forehead to Knee Position (Knee-Kiss Position)

Supine, Forehead to Knee Position (Knee-Kiss Position), will cause pain in the low-back area if tension is already present on a nerve root, as extra stretching is present because of cervical flexion.

Hip Range of Motion

The hip range of motion should always be checked for pain as well as movement and flexibility, as many times hip pathology is confused for low-back pain.

PAIN ASSESSMENT (1)

When did it start? Was it associated with injury? What other treatment have you had?

These questions will give the therapist insight into whether or not the back pain was associated with trauma, in which case a contusion, torn muscle, triggerpoint, or strain of the posterior joint might be the cause of pain. What other type of treatment the patient received will reveal other facts, like what type of treatment the pain did not respond to. From this information the therapist can usually use the process of elimination in further understanding of the pain. For example, if the back pain was believed to be originally from muscle trauma, and the patient received 1 month of therapy, 3 months ago, and still complains of pain, the therapist would probably suspect adhesions, a skeletal sprain, or a triggerpoint rather than the original trauma as the etiology of pain.

When is it Aggravated?

Mechanical pain is aggravated by movement and made worse by coughing. Usually it is better with rest. This type of pain is usually typical of a herniated intervertebral disc or stress fracture of a transverse process. Any movement that requires forward flexion, such as coming to a standing position, will intensify pain caused by a prolapsed intervertebral disc. However, extension and lateral flexion usually will not be affected. Pain arising from the spine, then, is influenced by posture, coughing, sneezing, and movement.

What Kind of Pain?

Referred pain, in contrast to pain intrinsic to the spine, is unrelated to movement, posture, or coughing. It is usually unremitting and colicky in nature and is not relieved by lying still. This type of pain may be referred from the pelvic or abdominal viscera. Pain arising from a woman's pelvic organs will often be described as pain similar to her period pain, but worse. Radiating pain, on the other hand, usually follows a dermatonal pattern, such as, along the sciatica, whereas referred pain does not. Seldom is referred pain felt below the knee, whereas radiating pain continues down into the calf or even the foot, following the nerve distribution.* Patients who awake early in the morning with unusual stiffness are usually suffering from an inflammatory disease, such as tuberculosis or ankylosing spondylitis. On the other hand, unremitting, excruciating pain is seldom caused by any back problem, even an acute herniated disc. If these are the presenting symptoms, more serious etiologies, such as metastasis to the spine and severe psychological problems, should be ruled out by the physician.

Which Activities Have Been Excluded by the Patient Because of Pain?

This information will provide the therapist with an accurate digest of which functional activities and movements cause pain and discomfort. Most times it will be more accurate than any other description of the patient's pain. These limitations will also form an important part of the patient's long-term goals.

Bowel or Bladder Problems?

If the patient presents with bowel or bladder paralysis, it could be symptomatic of the cauda equina syndrome or a massive herniation at a higher level, and should be reported to the physician immediately. This is often one of the indications for laminectomy.

Where is the Pain?

This diagram should be filled in by the therapist at the end of the assessment, except for the description of the patient's pain, which

---

*A severe sprain of the postfacet joint can cause both referred and radiating pain. The pain is usually referred into the low-back area, greater trochanter, and then radiates down the posterior lateral portion of the thigh, and sometimes into the leg and foot.

should be filled in at the beginning of the interview. The data recorded should not be limited to those categories listed in the lower left-hand corner. Everything of importance should be included, such as numbness, tingling, radiating pain, tenderness, etc. The area can be shaded and labeled to represent whatever the therapist wants to represent. The diagram should represent the results of the patient's assessment in a schematic form.

SUMMARY

The model on page 51 should represent both the patient's pain and symptom complaints, as compiled from the preceding pages of the patient's assessment. It should be the working model from which the physician will make his diagnosis, and the one from which the therapist constructs the treatment plan. Examples are given in Chap. 5.

It is evident from this type of logic that there is no standard type of back treatment that can successfully be applied to all patients. Hence, the days of the hot pack and five standard exercises are gone. Instead, the therapist is provided with a complete, organized, detailed evaluation procedure from which to identify the patient's limitations. Chap. 4 will provide treatment components from which the therapist will draw on to correct those limitations in a logical, systematic manner.

BIBLIOGRAPHY

Adams, J. (1973). *Outline of Orthopaedics.* Churchill, Livingstone, London.
Caillet, R. (1968). *Low Back Syndrome.* Davis, Philadelphia.
Farfan, H., and Lamy, B. (1977). A mathematical model of the soft tissue mechanisms of the lumbar spine. *Approaches to Validation of Manipulative Therapy.* A. A. Buerger and J. S. Tubis (Eds.). Thomas, Springfield, Ill.
Feinstein, B. (1977). Referred pain from paravertebral structures, approaches to validation of manipulation therapy.
Hoppenfield, S. (1977). *Physical Examination of the Spine and Extremities.* Appleton-Century-Crofts. New York.
Jayson, M. (Ed.) (1976). *The Lumbar Spine and Back Pain.* Sector Publishing Ltd., London.
Kraus H., (1952). Diagnosis and treatment of low back pain. *General Practitioner* V(4).
Kraus, H. (1970). *Clinical Treatment of Back and Neck Pain.* McGraw-Hill, New York.
Mcnab, I. (1977). *Backache.* Williams & Wilkins, Baltimore.

Magora, A., (1976). Conservative treatment of spondylolthises. *Clin Orthop*, Number 117.
Manual of Orthopaedic Surgery (1972). Published by the American Orthopaedic Association.
Mennell, J., and Zohn, D. (1976). *Diagnosis and Treatment of Musculoskeletal Pain*. Little, Brown, and Co., Boston.
Mooney, V., and Robertson, J. (1975). The facet syndrome. *Clin Orthop*, Number 115.
Nachemson, A. (1976). The lumbar spine, an Orthopaedic challenge. *Spine* 1(1).
Paine, K. (1975). Clinical features of lumbar spinal stenosis. *Clin Orthop*, Number 115.
Rosenberg, N. (1976). Degenerative spondylolisthesis. *Clin Orthop*, Number 117.
Williams, W. (1976). *Therapeutic Exercise for Body Alignment and Function*. Saunders, Philadelphia.

Chapter 4

A Complete Low-Back Exercise Program

This chapter represents a complete Low-Back Exercise Program as instituted at the New York Hospital at Cornell Medical Center. It outlines the physician's, as well as the therapist's, responsibilities in a hospital situation. However, the entire program is applicable by a therapist in private practice, or by an M.D. who treats low-back patients, and does not have the advantage of a skilled therapist to treat his or her patients.

Pages 66 to 70 explain the program and delineate responsibilities. Pages 71 to 131 are available as hand-outs to the patient at the therapist's discretion.

INTRODUCTION TO THE LOW-BACK EXERCISE PROGRAM

The purpose of this program is to systematically progress a patient's treatment from the painful acute stage to the point where he can perform a sound exercise program daily in a pain-free manner. This program is also designed to educate the patient by teaching him a functional approach to handling his/her back pain.

Each patient will have an exercise program designed specifically for him/her. The exercises will be carried out in a slow graduated manner determined by findings upon periodic reexaminations. At such times his/her program will be checked and progressed as necessary.

The M.D. should pinpoint the patient's specific problems. The therapist should be furnished with the following information: patient's occupation, physical activities, hobbies, neurological status, structural limitations and/or pathologies, whether it is a new injury or exacerbation of an existing condition.

A Complete Low-Back Exercise Program

The *therapist* will perform a flexibility examination, functional and manual muscle test, and a pain assessment on each patient.

There will be a bank of exercises from which the therapist will select specific ones based on the M.D.'s prescription.

The exercises will be grouped in the following categories:

1. Relaxation (R)
2. Limbering exercises (L)
3. Pelvic tilt exercises (P)
4. Low-back extensor stretching exercises (LBS)
5. Hip abductor strengthening exercises (HAS)
6. Hip extensor strengthening exercises (HES)
7. Hamstring stretching exercises (HS)
8. Hip flexor stretching exercises (HFS)
9. Abdominal strengthening exercises (AS)
10. Upper- and lower-back extensor strengthening exercises (BES)
11. Tensor fasciae latae stretching exercises (TFL)
12. Hip adductor stretching exercises (HAdS)

Progression of the patient's program to the more difficult exercises will be done by the therapist in consultation with the M.D.

The therapist will also teach the patient a program of correct body mechanics to facilitate his activities of daily living.

INFORMATION NEEDED FROM THE PHYSICIAN BEFORE COMMENCING THERAPY

History

Taken on initial M.D. examination.

> Chief complaint: history of present episode.
>
> Previous past episodes: when, what happened, treatment given.

Past health history (both personal and familial): illnesses, operations, etc. (if relevant to present condition).

Occupational history: type of work (heavy, light, sedentary).

Social history: especially if it brings tension or physical strain.

Medical summary: medications, allergies, endocrine history, other joint/muscle complaints, other complaints in general.

Psychological impression: depressed, anxious, nervous, other.

Pain history: location, radiation, related to activity or rest, what relieves it, medication, previous treatment, modalities, any previous treatment (chiropractor, etc.).

Clinical Examination

Done on initial and follow-up M.D. examination.

Gross flexibility test.

Posture profile.

Gross muscle test.

Palpation: spasms, triggerpoints, fibrositis.

Neurological tests: reflexes, sensation, etc.

X-ray review.

Referrals to Other Medical Specialists (if necessary)

Neurologic, endocrine, psychiatric, medical, other.

Impression

Differential diagnosis: disc, radiculopathy, R/O HNP, any general pathology or skeletal deformity, etc.

Initial diagnosis: low-back sprain, strain, radiculopathy, tension, muscle deficiency, muscle spasm, triggerpoint, etc.

Rehabilitation goal: symptomatic pain relief, decrease muscle spasm, relaxation, improve muscle strength or flexibility, etc.

Treatment plan:

1. For an acute muscle spasm, the program will consist of
   a. Medoclator, using a slowly increasing tetanizing current for 10 minutes and a surging current for 10 minutes.
   b. Ice or ethyl chloride (except when contraindicated).
   c. Relaxation (including passive ROM of neck—rotation, flexors, and extensors).
   d. Limbering exercise (including, if appropriate, LBS6).
   e. Explanation of theory and review of all written material.
   f. Instruction in home treatment program and ADL.

2. The three postinjection treatments will consist *only* of
   a. Medcolator, using a surging current for 15 minutes.
   b. Ice or ethyl chloride (except when contraindicated).
   c. Relaxation (including passive ROM of neck—rotation, flexors, and extensors).
   d. Limbering exercises.
   e. Explanation of theory and review of all written material.
   f. Instruction in home treatment and ADL.

3. The therapist will select the appropriate exercises based upon the physician's assessment that it is an acute or chronic condition and also based on the M.D.'s and therapist's evaluation. Progression of exercises from acute to maintenance-oriented will also be done in consultation with the physician.

   In addition, an analysis of job- and home-related postural habits, e.g., sitting, standing, walking posture, athletic activities, etc., will also be evaluated.

4. The therapist will select the appropriate exercises based upon the physician's assessment that it is an acute or chronic condition. Progression of exercises from acute to maintenance-oriented will also be done in consultation with the physician.

5. Each exercise will be taught in exactly the same way by each therapist. There will be *no modification* of individual exercise, and only the listed exercises will be used.

6. The therapist will keep an accurate and current record of all exercises that have been given to each patient. This must be done both on the patient's take home sheet and in the departmental records.

7. General relaxation regime will be given only when specifically ordered by the M.D. If the therapist feels it would be beneficial, they should consult with the patient's physician.

8. The therapist will carefully review with the patient all written material handed to him/her in order to ensure

   a. that the patient has a clear understanding of the need for an exercise program;

   b. that the patient understands the theory underlying the treatment;

   c. that the patient clearly understands all the instructions.

The New York Hospital-Cornell Medical Center Department of Rehabilitation Medicine
Questions and Answers About Your Low-Back Condition

HOW TO GET RID OF BACK PAIN CAUSED BY TIGHT MUSCLES

The first aim of your exercise program is to relax your muscles. When muscles are contracted for too long a time or too suddenly, they can go into a painful muscle spasm, when they will shorten. Therefore, one goal of your back program will be to remove excess tension from your muscles and constantly attempt to return your back muscles to the length of their normal "resting state."

WHAT CAUSES A MUSCLE TO GO INTO SPASM?

Postural strain—standing, sitting, driving, or holding any position for too long a time.

Sudden changes—from overwork/underwork and vice versa, put a strain on the muscles.

Emotional tension—has a cumulative effect on your vulnerable skeletal muscles, i.e., back and neck muscles.

Trauma—the body automatically reacts to injury by tensing up the muscles around the injured part. The same applies when a nerve is irritated by pressure or inflammation.

Stress—when we are presented with a threatening situation, normal body defenses are alerted for action and, if these actions are supressed for any reason, there is a build-up of tension in the voluntary muscles. This may lead to painful muscle spasm.

Triggerpoints—some groups of muscle fibers that were subjected to strain or injury do not relax in spite of exercises. These stay "clumped up" and are sometimes the focus of pain. These triggerpoints can be felt on examination as firm nodes, painful to pressure. Your doctor will discuss their treatment with you.

WHY EXERCISE?

The exercises you receive at the beginning of your program may seem exceptionally simple to do. There should be no strain, stress, or fatigue involved. The goal of these exercises is only to return your muscles to their natural resting state.

Later on, you will receive an expanded program that will concentrate on strengthening your muscles, but you will always begin and end your program with those exercises designed to return your muscles to their natural resting state.

Exercise is the only way to create a balanced muscular system, and the only way to maintain it is to do the exercises every day. It must become as much a part of your daily life as brushing your teeth. It must become a habit.

WHAT WILL THE EXERCISES BE?

Your program will be given to you gradually, a few exercises at a time, by a physical therapist. It will see you through the acute phase until you have a complete program specifically designed to deal with your musculoskeletal problem. To benefit most from such a program, you must return for periodic reevaluation and reinstruction.

HOW LONG WILL YOU NEED TO DO EXERCISES?

Once you have had an episode of back pain, there is always the chance it can happen again. The best way to build up a defense against such low-back pain attack is to exercise every day for the indefinite future and to move your body using correct body mechanics.

Once developed, your individual exercise program should be used as a way to "warm up" and "cool down" before and after engaging in any sport. Your physical therapist will give you more information on how to fully incorporate your back program into your particular life style.

How to Perform the Exercise

Give yourself enough time to do the exercises. They must be done in a relaxed atmosphere, so it is important that you do not allow interruptions or distractions once you begin. Never do them when you are in a rush. You can do them at any time of the day except immediately after eating. The days when you are very rushed, under a lot of stress, or nervous, are the days that you need to do the exercises the most! Make a special effort to do them on these days.

In the beginning exercises, special attention should be placed on understanding the difference between the two phases of each exercise. The first phase is the tightening and the second is the letting go. This second phase, the "letting go," is equally important. It helps you to learn to feel the difference between a tense muscle and a relaxed muscle.

Do the exercises in the order they were given to you by your therapist and do the number of repetitions prescribed. Your exercise program should always begin and end with the simple limbering exercises. To obtain maximum benefit from your exercise program, start with the first exercise and do all of the exercises the prescribed number of times. After you have done the last exercise, reverse the program by starting with the second to the last exercise and proceed until you have worked backward to the very first exercise (deep breathing).

Do the exercises slowly and smoothly on a hard surface. Get onto a carpeted floor if necessary. You may place a small pillow under your head if you wish. Relax for a few seconds between *each* exercise. Wear comfortable loose clothing. NEVER hold your breath while exercising. If you find that you continue to hold your breath, count out loud or make some effort to breathe out.

Do only the exercise program given to you by your therapist. These exercises should not cause increased pain. If they do, stop doing them and report it to your therapist or physician.

If you are engaged in any other exercise programs, please inform the physician and the therapist.

Your Home Treatment

Adequate treatment of an acute muscle spasm requires attention several times a day. Therefore, in order to augment the physical therapy treatment you receive at The New York Hospital, we are supplying you with the following instructions for the Ice Massage and exercise.

WHY IS ICE USED IN YOUR THERAPY PROGRAM?

When a muscle is in a shortened state and painful, it influences nerves in the area and the muscle can go into spasm (a painful contraction). Ice is used so we can return the muscle to its natural resting state without causing more pain, which will lead to more spasm, etc. It is a vicious cycle that we can break with ice.

ICE MASSAGE

Fill 4 oz. paper cup three-quarters full and put in freezer until frozen.

When ready to use, tear off about one inch of the cup so that some of the ice is showing while the bottom of the cup can be used to hold onto.

Massage the entire muscle area as instructed by your therapist. You may use circular or up and down strokes, but do *not* hold the ice in one spot.

THERE ARE FOUR PHASES TO THE ICE MASSAGE:

1. Cold   which you feel when you first apply the ice
2. Ache   after a few minutes

3.	Burning	after about 5 minutes it will feel like your skin is burning. At this point, remove the ice for a minute or so.
4.	Numbness	THIS IS THE CRUCIAL PHASE. Return the ice and massage until all the burning disappears. This signals the end of the ice massage.

Now the ice massage is completed. The entire procedure should take 5 to 7 minutes. Do *not* massage more than 7 minutes for a small area or more than 10 minutes for a large area.

An alternative to this method is to use a plastic bag filled with ice cubes. Wrap ice-filled plastic bag in a thin wet towel and place it over area indicated by the therapist. Keep in place for 20-30 minutes following criteria listed above under four phases to ice massage.

EXERCISE

Now you can very gently stretch the tender muscle by following the exercises prescribed by your therapist. Do not perform any sudden, jerky movement, or do more exercises than the number and repetitions given to you. Should you feel any pain while exercising, use the ice for another minute or two, until the pain disappears. You should feel no pain while exercising.

Repeat this procedure three times (3X) a day.

General Relaxation

Lie on your back on a hard surface with one or two pillows under your knees. Close your eyes.

Perform the deep breathing exercises taught you previously.

Wobble head a few times.

Squeeze your eyes shut as tightly as possible. Let the tightness go. Breathe.

Squeeze all of your face muscles together. Let the tightness go. Breathe.

Squeeze your lips together. Let go. Breathe.

Wobble head a few times.

Squeeze your shoulder blades together. Let go.

Tighten your chest muscles by rounding your shoulders. Let go. Breathe.

Pull in your stomach muscles. Let go.

Tighten your buttocks. Let go.

Push the small of your back into the floor. Let go. Breathe.

Make a fist with the right hand as tight as possible. Let go.

Repeat with left hand. Let go. Breathe.

Bend the right hand at the elbow and let it sway back and forth. Imagine your entire body being as light and as free as your hand. Breathe.

Repeat with the left hand. Let your whole body be light and free and loose. Breathe.

Slide your right leg out as far as it will go. Push it into the pillow. Let go. Squeeze the toes together. Let go. Wobble the leg. Breathe. Return the leg to the bent knee position.

Repeat on left leg.

To finish the exercise, open your eyes, and stretch your arms overhead and your legs in the opposite direction, similar to a yawning stretch.

A Complete Low-Back Exercise Program

RELAXATION

To precede EACH exercise session. Lie on your back with one or two pillows under your knees.

R1 BREATHING

Inhale through your nose. Blow out slowly and gently through pursed lips. Repeat _____ times.

R2 HEAD WOBBLE

Gently roll your head from side to side a few times until you feel relaxed. The head should be allowed to drop to each side using no muscular effort to hold it in any one position.

R3 SHOULDER SHRUG

Bring your shoulders up toward your ears and then let them drop completely. Repeat _____ times.

L1 KNEE TO CHEST - BACK-LYING

Lie on your back with knees bent and feet flat on mat.

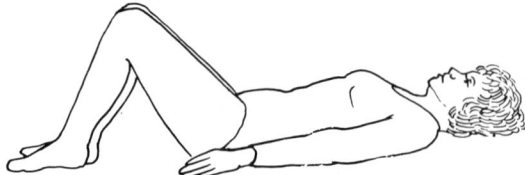

Raise the right knee up to your chest as far as possible without straining or using your hands, and then return the foot to the floor with the knee bent.

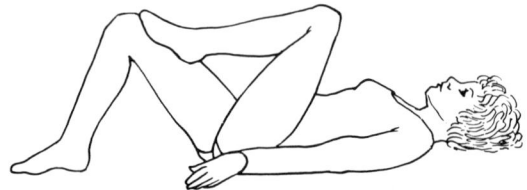

Slide the heel out along the mat until the leg is straight. Gently roll the leg from side to side. Return to starting position. Repeat with other leg.

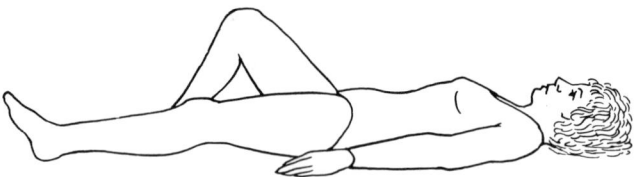

Repeat _____ times with each leg.

A Complete Low-Back Exercise Program 81

L2 KNEE TO CHEST - SIDE-LYING

Lie on your right side, with knees slightly bent up toward your chest. Place pillow under your head.

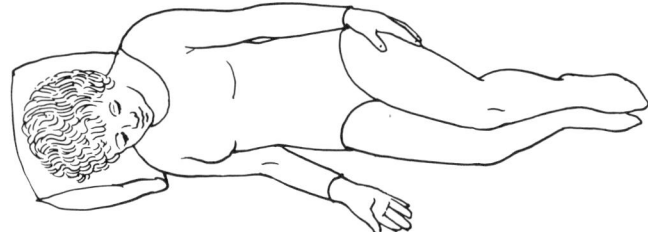

Slide your left knee up to your chest without straining. At this point drop the knee onto the floor.

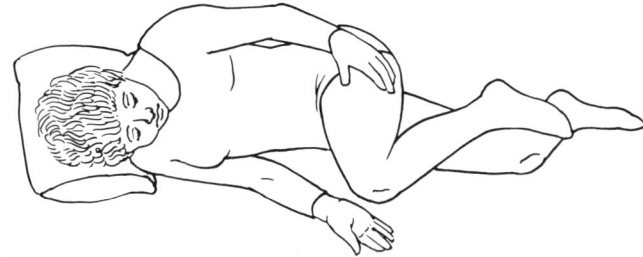

Then gently straighten out the leg so that both the hip and knee are straight. Again, drop the leg to the floor so that no effort is used to hold it. Return the leg to the starting position.

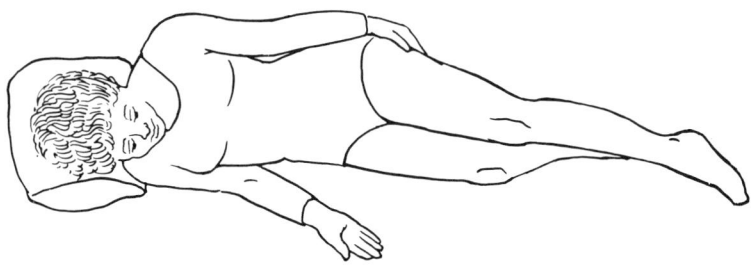

Repeat _____ times. Turn onto your left side and repeat the exercise _____ times.

L3 BUTTOCKS PINCH - ON YOUR STOMACH

Roll onto your stomach and if instructed by your therapist put a pillow under your stomach. Squeeze your buttocks together tightly and LET GO.

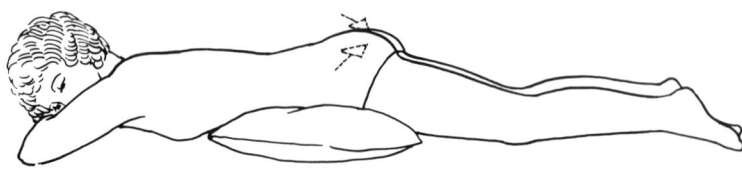

Repeat _____ times.

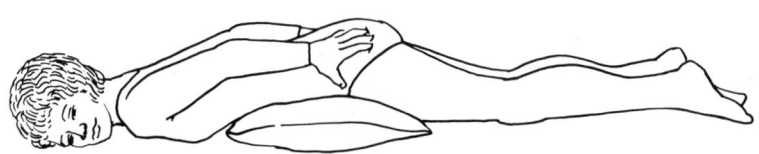

(If you have difficulty doing this movement, place one hand on each buttock, and gently squeeze them together until you can do it without your hands.)

NOTE

Your physical therapy treatments are carefully planned for optimum results. It is imperative, therefore, that you perform your exercises both at home, and in the hospital, in a particular order.

Always start your program with No. _____ and go all the way through to No. _____. Reverse the program by going back to No. _____ and return to the beginning, ending with No. _____.

In this manner, you will always begin and end your exercise session with the relaxation exercises and the deep breathing.

NOTE:

If you have received an injection by your doctor, your three post-injection physical therapy treatments are carefully planned for optimum results. It is imperative, therefore, that you perform your exercises both at home, and in the hospital, in a particular order.

Always start your program with No. _____ and go all the way through to No. _____. Reverse the program by going back to No. _____ and return to the beginning, ending with No. _____.

In this manner, you will always begin and end your exercise session with the relaxation exercises and the deep breathing.

P1 PELVIC TILT - BACK-LYING

Lie on your back with knees bent and feet flat on the mat. Keep your arms at your side.

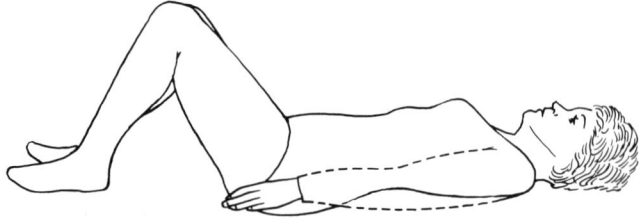

Push the small of your back into the mat, by pinching your buttocks together and pulling in your stomach, until it is flat against the mat. Count out loud to _____. Let go.

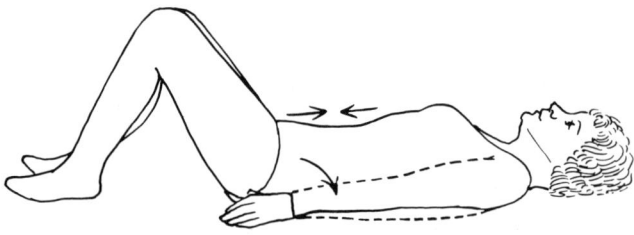

Repeat _____ times

A Complete Low-Back Exercise Program

P2 PELVIC TILT - SITTING

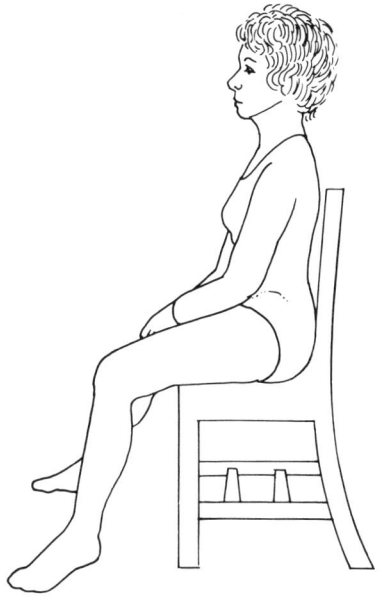

Sit in a straight back chair with your feet flat on the floor. Relax against the back of your chair.

Pull in your stomach muscles, squeeze your buttocks together and try to push the small of your back down and into the back of the chair. Count out loud to _____.
Let go.

Repeat _____ times.

P3 PELVIC TILT - STANDING

Standing with your back and shoulder blades against the wall, feet should be about eight inches from the wall, knees are slightly bent. In this position do a pelvic tilt until the small of your back is flat against the wall. Count out loud to _____. Let go.

Repeat _____ times.

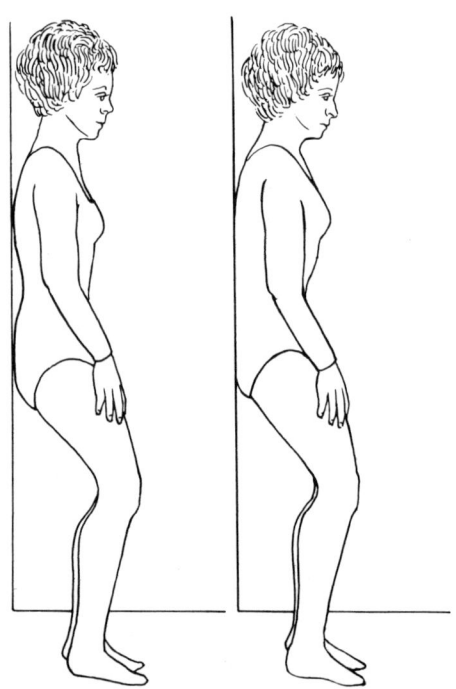
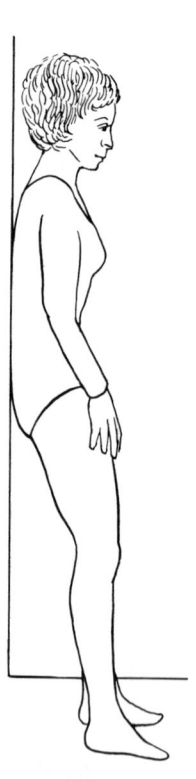

a. Follow above instructions, but maintain the pelvic tilt as you straighten your knees, and then count out loud to six. Let go.

  Repeat _____ times

P4 PELVIC TILT - BACK-LYING

Lie on your back and assume pelvic tilt position. Maintain tilt as you straighten your knees by slowly sliding your heels along the surface. Stop when you are no longer able to hold a full tilt position (about half-way). Hold there and count out loud to six.

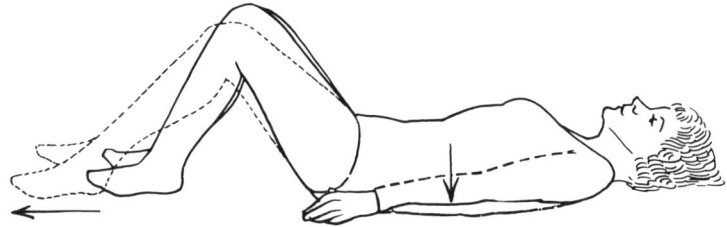

a. After holding six seconds, first bring one leg and then the other back to the starting position maintaining pelvic tilt throughout. Let go.

b. After holding for six seconds, slide both legs simultaneously back to the starting position maintaining pelvic tilt throughout. Let go.

Repeat _____ times.

LBS1 LOW BACK EXTENSOR STRETCHING - ON HANDS AND KNEES

Assume a hands-and-knees position, with your hands underneath your shoulders, and knees shoulder-width apart. Do not bend your elbows throughout the entire exercise.

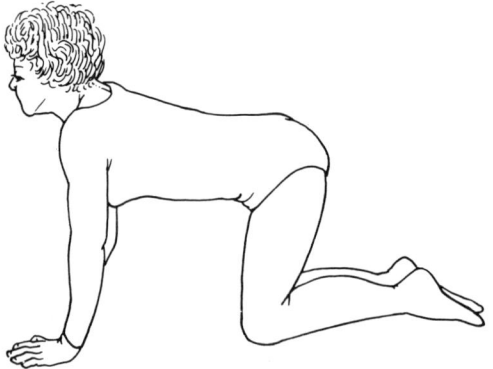

Drop your head, pull in your stomach muscles, and try to get your back as round and as high as possible.

Exhale while assuming this position to the count of _____.

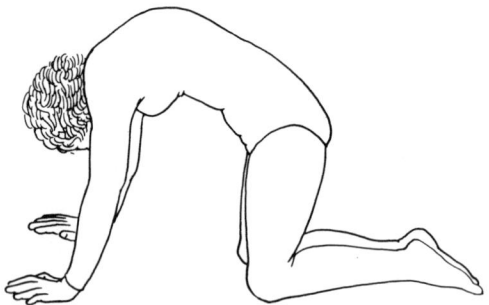

Now, raise your head up and relax your back, returning to starting position. Inhale while assuming this position. Hold to the count of

Repeat this entire exercise _____ times.

A Complete Low-Back Exercise Program 89

LBS2 LOW BACK EXTENSOR STRETCHING - BACK-LYING

Lie on your back with your arms at your sides.

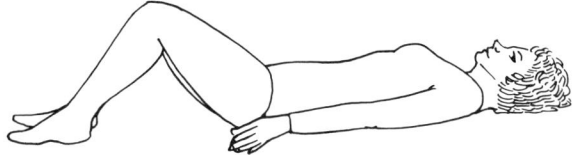

Begin to exhale slowly while you lift your head. Lift up only far enough so that you can see your navel. Exhale by counting out loud to _____.

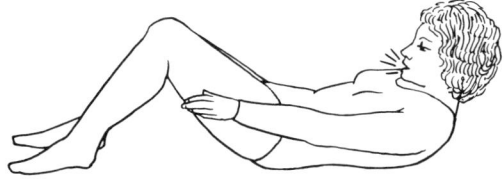

Return to the floor, gently roll your head from side to side.

Repeat _____ times.

LBS3 LOW BACK EXTENSOR STRETCHING - BACK-LYING

Lie on your back, with feet flat on the floor and both knees bent.

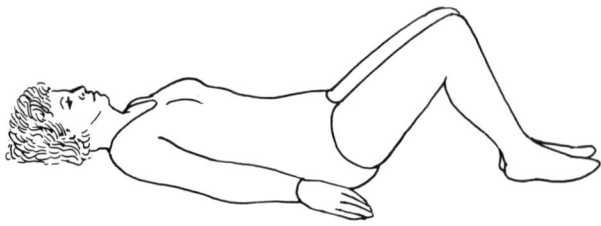

Bring your right knee up toward your chest, without straining or using your hands.

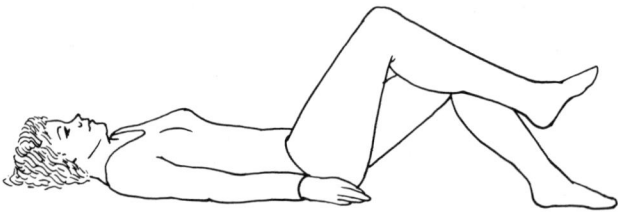

Begin to exhale slowly and lift your head, trying to touch your forehead to your knee. Do not strain. Hold this position while you count to _____ .

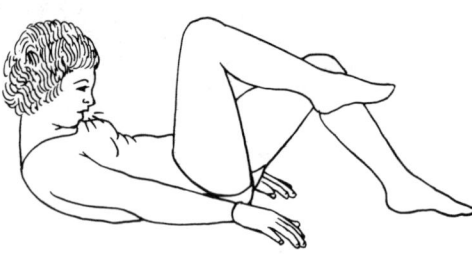

Return your head and then your right foot to the floor. Roll your head gently from side to side. Repeat with the left leg.

Repeat _____ times with each leg.

LBS4 LOW BACK EXTENSOR STRETCHING - BACK-LYING

Lie on your back, with your knees bent and feet flat on the floor.

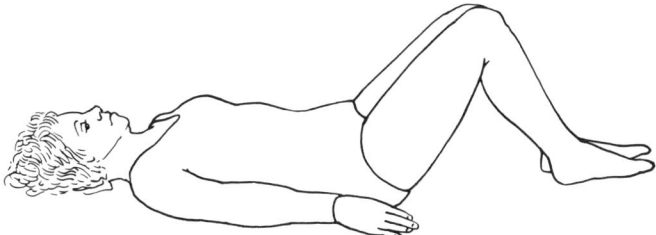

Bring both knees up to your chest and gently grasp them with your arms.

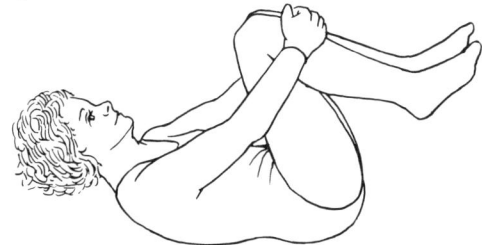

Exhale slowly while you lift your head off the floor toward your knees. Push knees away until elbows are fully extended. The movement should take to the count of six.

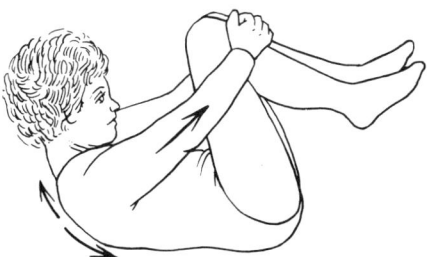

Return your head and then your feet to the floor. Gently roll your head from side to side, inhale, and repeat _____ times.

LBS5 LOW BACK EXTENSOR STRETCHING WITH ROTATION - BACK-LYING

Lie on your back, with your knees bent and feet flat on the mat.

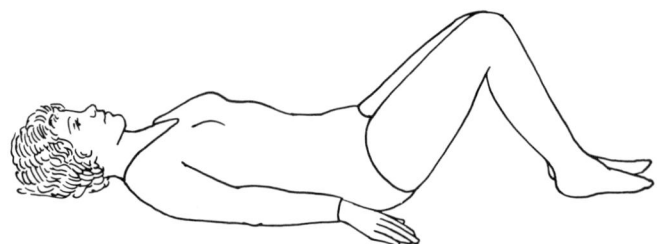

Bring both knees up to your chest without using your hands. This motion should cause the small of your back to be level with the mat (pelvic tilt).

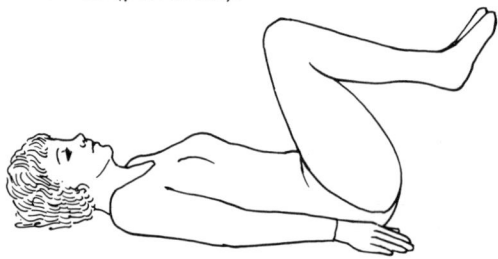

Gently drop both knees to the right, and let them rest completely on the mat for _____ seconds. Make sure your shoulders remain on the mat throughout the exercise.

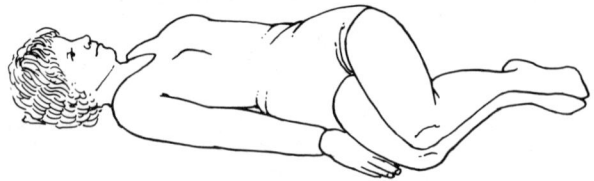

Return your knees to your chest and drop them to the left for _____ seconds.

Return to the bent-knee position, feet flat on the mat.

Repeat _____ times to each side.

LBS6 LOW BACK EXTENSOR STRETCHING - SITTING

Sit in a straight-back chair, with your feet flat on the floor, knees spread shoulder-width apart. Let your hands hang loosely at your sides or between your knees. Tuck your chin on your chest.

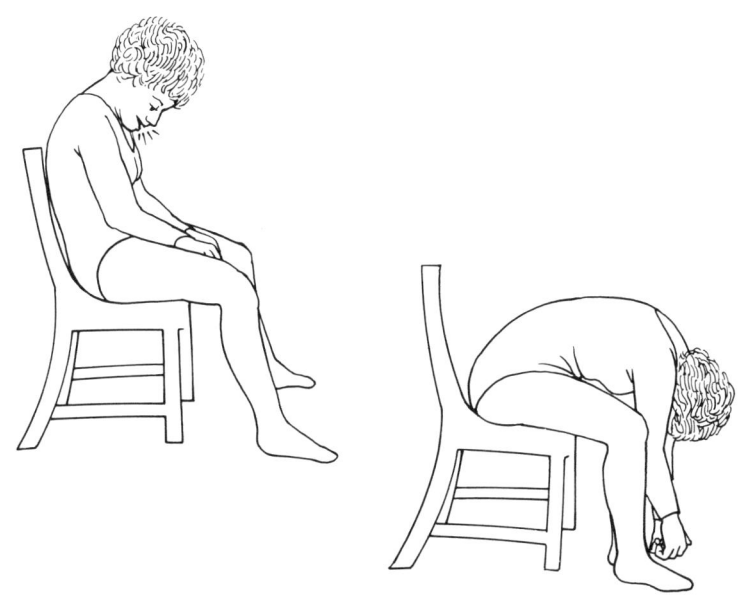

Drop your shoulders, and roll down so that your arms are dangling on the floor. Do not force yourself down to touch the floor, or do any jerky or bouncing movement.

Retain this position for _____ seconds.

Return to the sitting position by tightening the abdominal muscles and squeezing your buttocks.

Continue to roll up first the lower back, then the shoulders and finally, the head.

Exhale while rolling down, inhale while rolling up.

Repeat _____ times.

LBS7 LOW BACK EXTENSOR STRETCHING WITH ROTATION - SITTING

Sit in a straight-back chair, with your feet flat on the floor, and knees spread shoulder-width apart. Turn your body slightly to the left and let both hands hang loosely over your left knee.

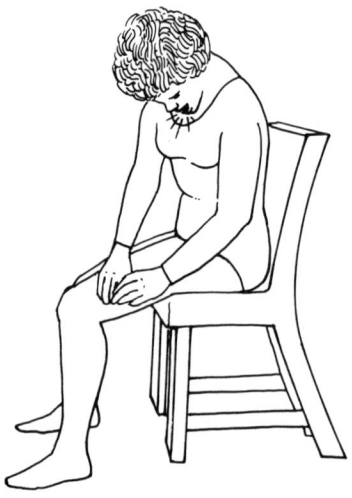

Tuck your chin on you chest, drop your shoulders, and roll down so that your arms are dropping toward the floor, and your right shoulder is near your left knee. Do not force yourself down to touch the floor, and do not do any jerky or bouncing movements.

Retain this position for _____ seconds.

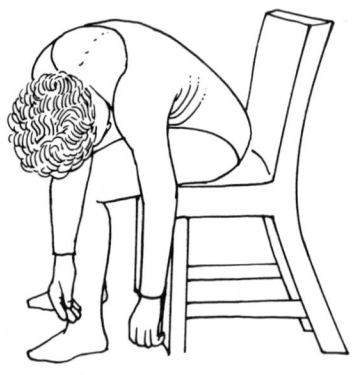

Return to the sitting position by tightening the abdominal muscles and squeezing your buttocks. Continue to roll up first the lower back, then the shoulders and, finally, the head.

Exhale while rolling down, inhale while rolling up.
Repeat to the right side

Repeat _____ times to each side.

A Complete Low-Back Exercise Program

HAS1 HIP ABDUCTOR STRENGTHENING - BACK-LYING

Lie on your back with left leg outstretched and right leg bent with foot on the floor.

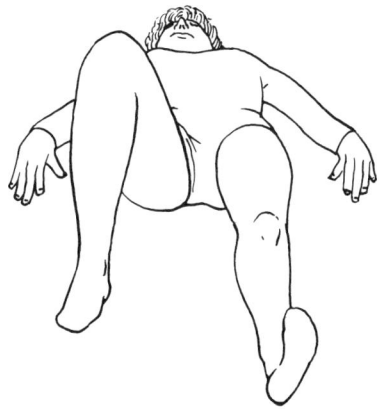

Slide the heel of the left foot along the mat toward your left as far as possible. Keep the knee straight and kneecap pointing to the ceiling. Hold it there for the count of six. Slide the heel back to the midline, roll it gently,

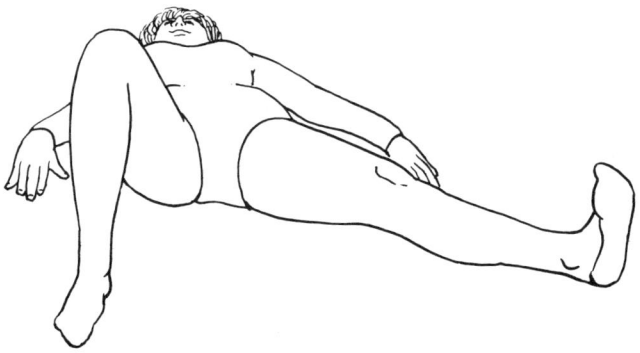

Repeat_____times with each leg.

HAS2 HIP ABDUCTOR STRENGTHENING - SIDE-LYING

Lie on your right side. The bottom leg may be slightly bent, but the top leg must be kept straight.

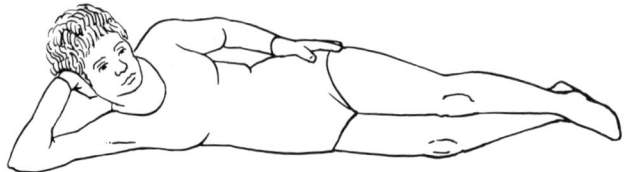

Slowly lift your left leg straight up toward the ceiling, as far as possible. Do not bend at the hip, either forward or backward. Keep the kneecap facing forward and leg in line with the body. Hold this position while counting out loud to six. Return it slowly and repeat _____ times.

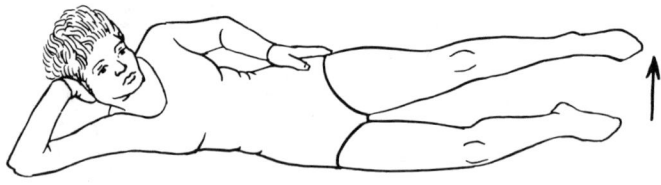

Lie on your left side and repeat exercise with right leg.

Repeat _____ times.

HES1 HIP EXTENSOR STRENGTHENING - STOMACH-LYING

Roll onto your stomach, and if instructed by your therapist, put a pillow under your stomach. Squeeze your buttocks together tightly, and count out loud to six. Let go.

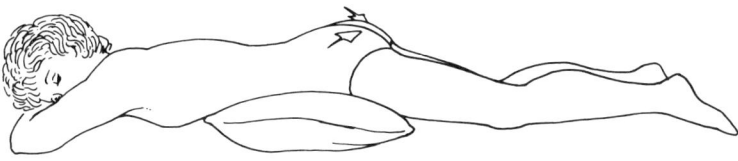

Repeat _____ times.

(If you have difficulty doing this movement, place one hand on each buttock, and gently squeeze them together until you can do it without your hands.)

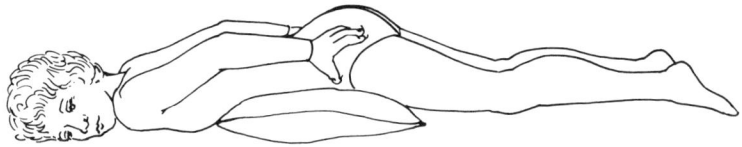

HES2 HIP EXTENSOR STRENGTHENING - STOMACH-lying

Roll onto your stomach, and if instructed by your therapist, put a pillow under your stomach.

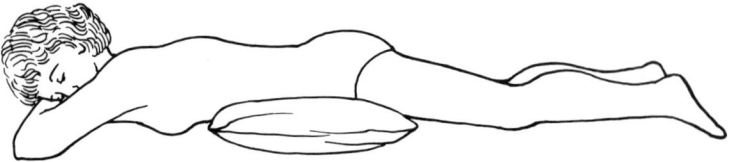

Bend your left knee so that the sole of your foot is facing the ceiling, and raise your left thigh up, off the mat as far as possible, keeping your pelvis flat on the mat. Count out loud to six, and return the leg to the floor. Straighten the knee, roll the leg gently, and repeat on the other side.

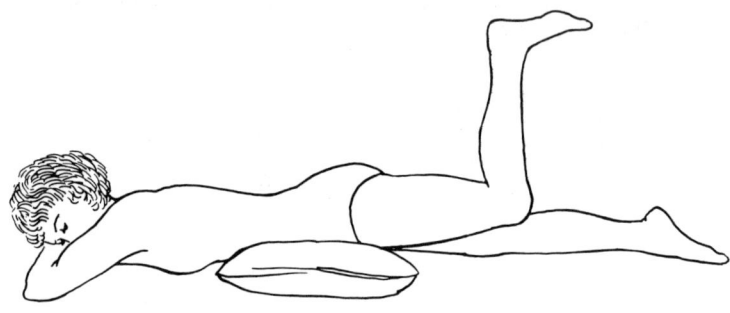

Repeat _____ times with each leg.

HES3 HIP EXTENSOR STRENGTHENING - BACK/LYING

Lie on your back, with two pillows under your knees. Keep feet flat. Use no pillow under your head.

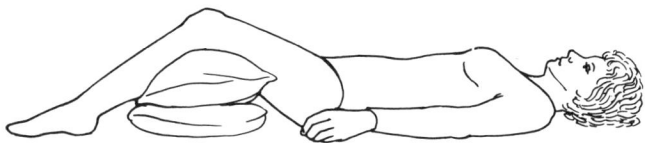

Push the back of your knees into the pillows and your shoulders into the floor so that your buttocks raise off the floor. Count out loud to six. Do not hold your breath. Return slowly to the floor. Let go of all tightness.

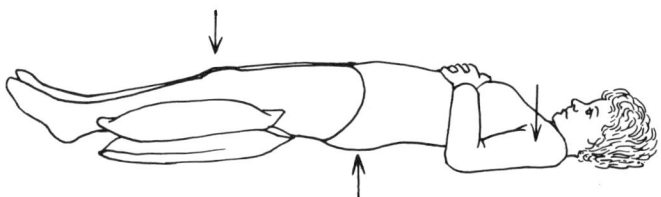

Repeat _____ times.

HES4 HIP EXTENSOR STRENGTHENING - BACK/LYING

Lie on your back with knees bent and feet flat on the mat. Use no pillow under your head.

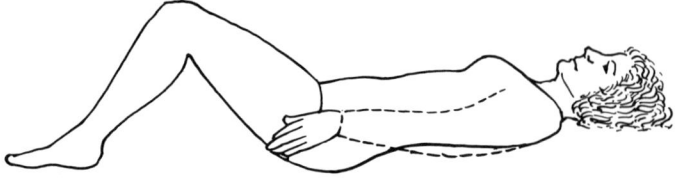

Push down and lift buttocks off the floor. Shoulders should remain on the floor. Count out loud to six. Return slowly to the floor. Let go.

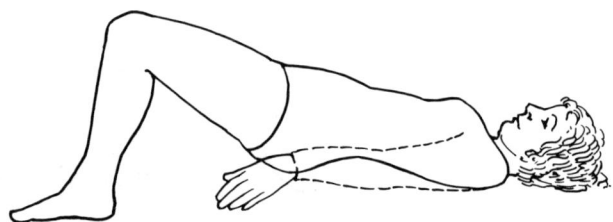

Repeat _____ times.

HS1 HAMSTRING STRETCHING - SITTING

Sit on the edge of a bed so that your left leg is straight out on the bed and your right leg is off the side resting on the floor or supported by a chair. On the left leg, bend the ankle up and straighten the knee. Hold for the count of _____.

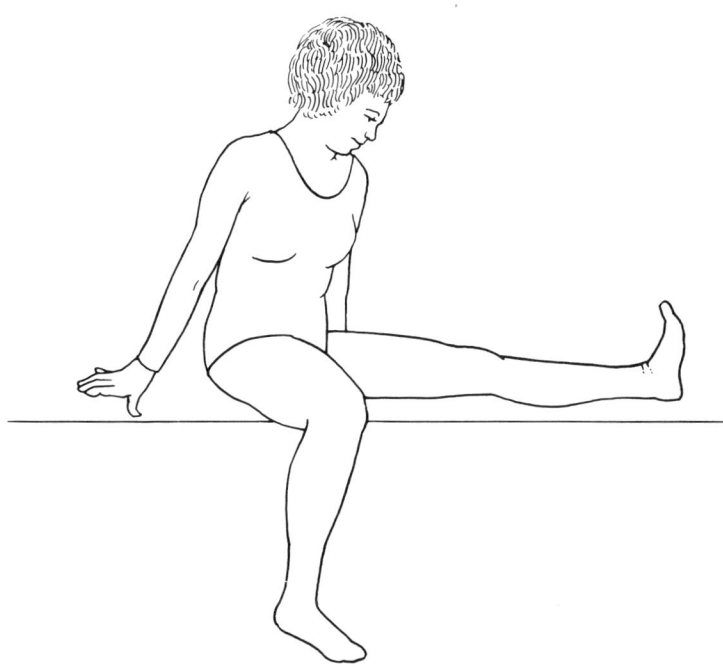

Roll the leg and bend the knee slightly between each exercise.

Repeat _____ times with left leg.   Change position and repeat with the right leg.

HS2 HAMSTRING STRETCHING - BACK-LYING

Lie on your back with both knees bent and feet flat on the floor.

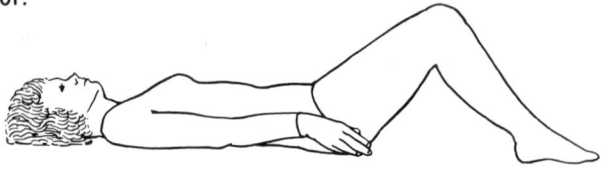

Bring your right knee to your chest.

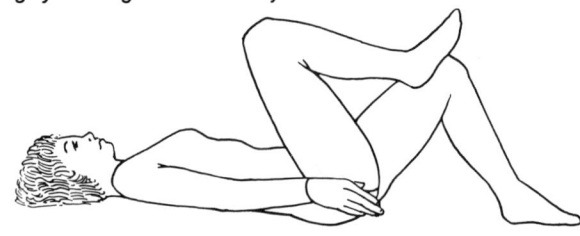

From this position, slowly straighten your leg toward the ceiling until your knee is straight. You may have to lower the leg to get the knee completely straight. Hold it there for the count of _____. Repeat _____ times with each leg.

Lower leg to the floor. Roll it from side to side and return to bent knee position.

b.

b. Assume bent knee position. Bring right knee to chest, bend ankle up and then straighten leg toward the ceiling attempting to achieve straight knee position. Follow above instructions.

Repeat _____ times with each leg.

HS3 HAMSTRING STRETCHING - BACK-LYING

Lie on your back, with feet flat on the floor and both knees bent.

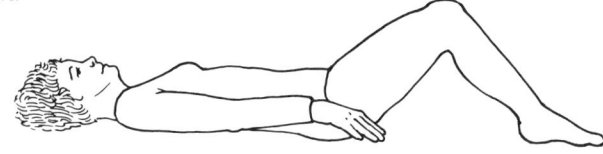

Push the small of your back into the floor (pelvic tilt), slide your right foot out until your leg is straight, bend your ankle up.

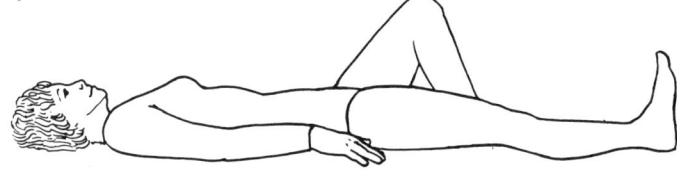

Slowly lift your leg straight up in the air. Make sure you keep your knee straight throughout the entire exercise.

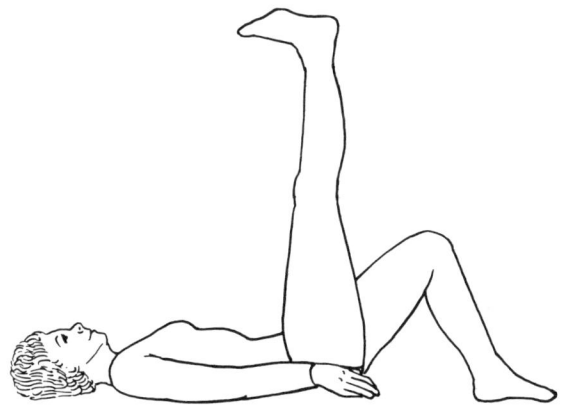

Raise the leg up until you feel a "pull" in the back of your thigh, and hold it there to the count of _____ . Lower your leg to the floor, roll it, and return to the bent knee position.

Repeat _____ times with each leg.

HS4 HAMSTRING STRETCHING - STANDING

Standing with your feet at shoulder-width, and arms relaxed at your side. Tuck your chin onto your chest, and roll down so that your hands are dangling toward the floor.

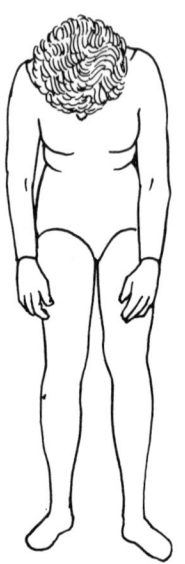

Keep your knees straight. Do not force yourself down to touch the floor, or do any jerky or bouncy movements. You should feel a "pull" in the lower back, and behind the thighs.

Hold this position for as long as comfortable, up to 15 seconds. Return to the standing position by rolling up, first the lower back, then the shoulders, and finally, the head.

Exhale while rolling down - Inhale while rolling up.

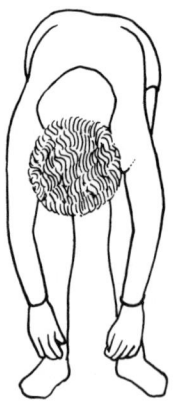

Repeat _____ times.

A Complete Low-Back Exercise Program

HS5 HAMSTRING STRETCHING - SITTING

Sit on the edge of a bed so that your right leg is out straight on the bed, and your left leg is on the floor or supported by a chair.

Bend the ankle up and straighten the knee of the right leg, and slowly bend over reaching toward your right knee. Hold this position for the count of 15. Do not bounce or jerk.

Roll the leg, and bend the knee slightly between each exercise.

(later reach toward your ankle)

Repeat _____ times with each leg.

Change your position and repeat with the left leg.

HS6 HAMSTRING STRETCHING - SITTING

Sit on the floor with your legs straight and spread in a "v" position.

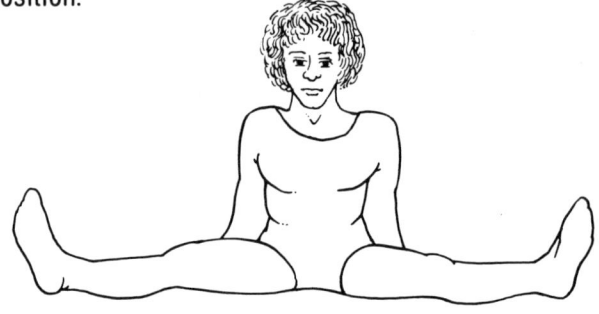

Bend your right ankle up, and while keeping the knee straight, gently bend over your right leg with your arms reaching toward your knee (later toward your ankle), and hold this position for 15 seconds. Do not bounce. Return to the sitting position, roll your right leg, and repeat over the left leg.

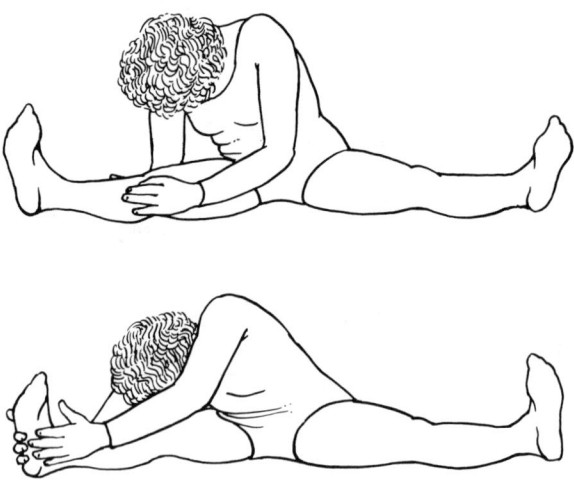

Repeat _____ times to each side.

HS7 hamstring stretching - SITTING

Sit on the floor with your legs outstretched before you. Cross your left leg over your right leg, and bend forward slowly.

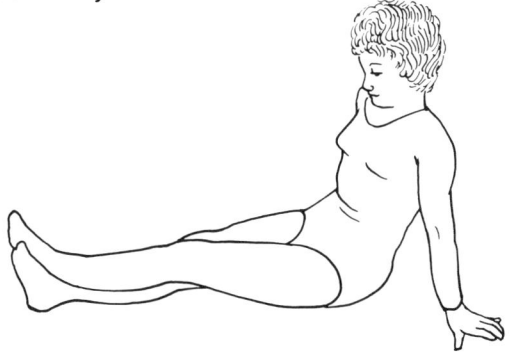

Reach forward toward your knee. Do not bounce or jerk. You should feel the pull on the underneath of the bottom leg. Hold this position for the count of 15.
Then return to starting position.

Repeat _____ times.

(later reach toward your ankle)
Repeat _____ times.

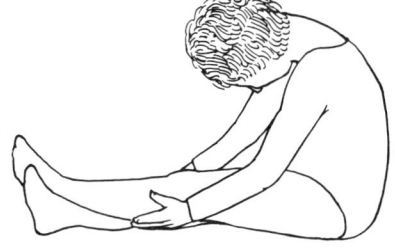

Then reverse and cross your right leg over your left leg and proceed as above.

Repeat _____ times.

HS8 HAMSTRING STRETCHING - STANDING

Keeping your knees bent, roll down so that you can hook your fingers underneath your toes.

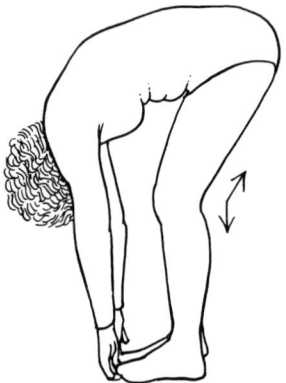

Slowly straighten your knees. Hold this position while counting out loud to six.

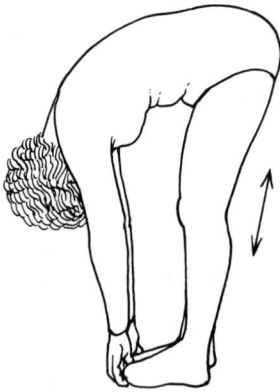

Bend your knees and repeat _____ times.

HFS1 HIP FLEXOR STRETCHING - BACK-LYING

Breathe out as you bring both knees toward chest.

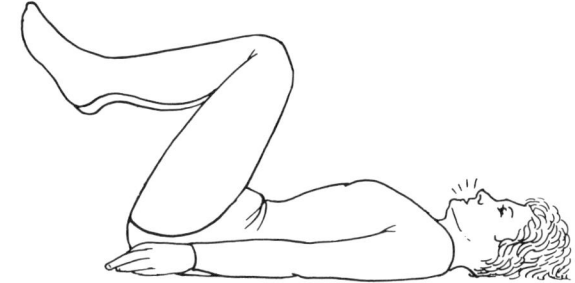

Hold one knee tightly to chest with arms. Slide other leg down until it is flat, trying to touch back of knee to the floor. Hold while you count out loud to six. Slowly return to the starting position. Relax. Alternate legs.

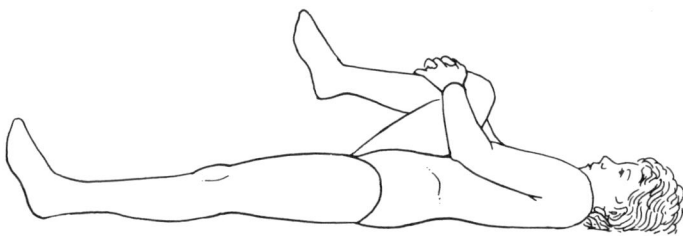

Repeat _____ times with each leg.

HFS2 HIP FLEXOR STRETCHING - BACK-LYING

Lie on bed for this exercise. Knees bent with feet at the foot of the bed. Bring one knee up to chest and hold it with your hands.

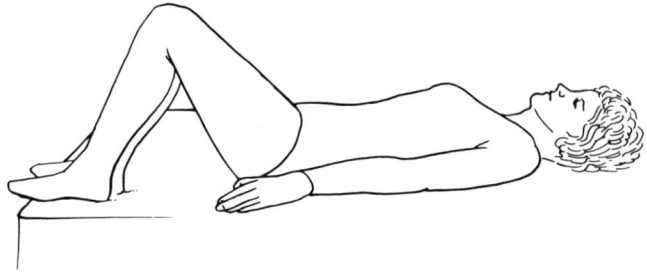

Lower the other leg so that the knee is bent over the foot of the bed and hanging free. Hold this position for 15 to 30 seconds. Return to starting position. Alternate legs.

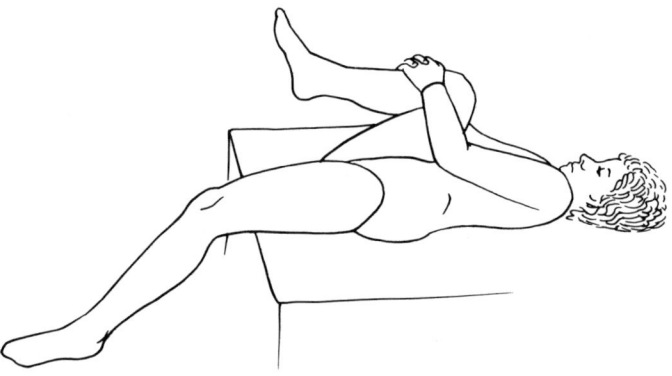

Repeat _____ times with each leg.

HFS3 HIP FLEXOR STRETCHING - BACK-LYING

Lie on your back close to the edge of the bed. Bend both knees up.

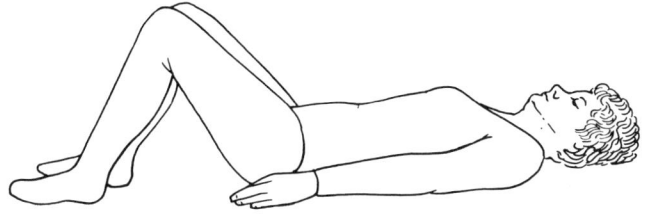

Bring inside leg up to chest and hold it with your hands.

Slide the outside leg out straight, over the edge, so that it will dangle at the level of mid-thigh. Hold this position for 15 to 30 seconds. Return both legs to the bent knee position.

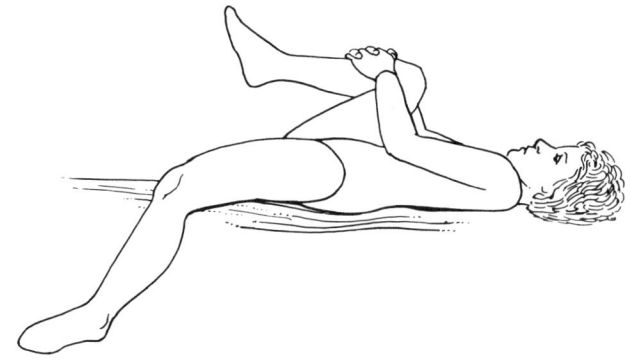

Repeat _____ times.

Change position and repeat on the alternate leg.

HFS4 HIP FLEXOR STRETCHING - SIDE-LYING

Lie on your right side and bring your left heel toward the left buttock. Keep bottom leg slightly bent.

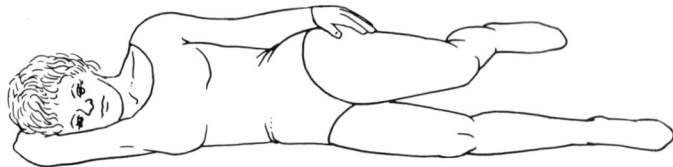

Grasp the top part of your left ankle with your hand and push the knee back, past the right leg. Do not arch your back. (you can prevent this by slightly bending forward at the waist before bringing the leg back.) Hold this position for 15 seconds.

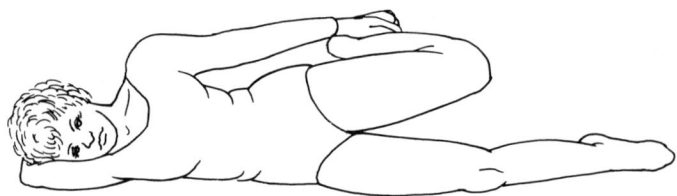

Repeat_____times with each leg.

AS1 ABDOMINAL STRENGTHENING - BACK-LYING

Lie on your back with knees bent and feet flat. Breathe in deeply, and forcefully blow out through pursed lips.

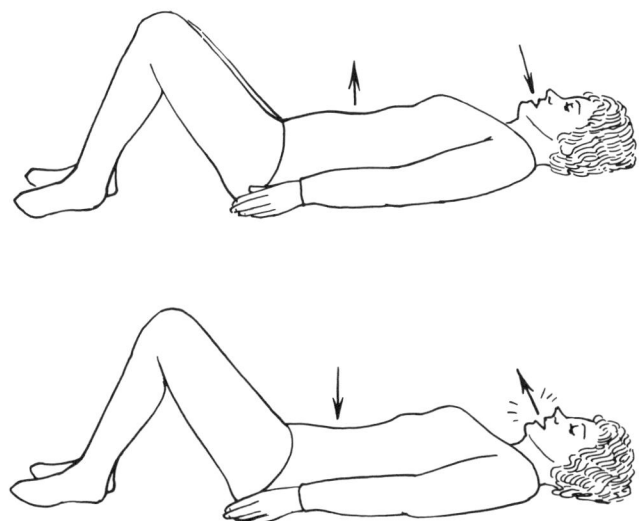

Pull in stomach muscles while blowing out. This forced exhalation should take approximately two seconds longer than the inhalation. Inhale and repeat _____ times.

AS2 ABDOMINAL STRENGTHENING - BACK-LYING

Lie on your back with knees bent and feet flat on the mat. Keep your arms at your side.

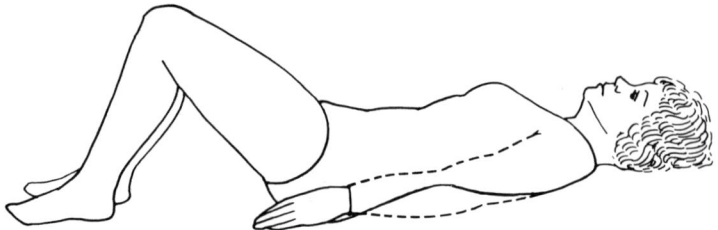

Push the small of your back into the floor by pinching your buttocks together and pulling in your stomach until it is flat against the floor. Breathe out as you do this by counting out loud to six. Let go.

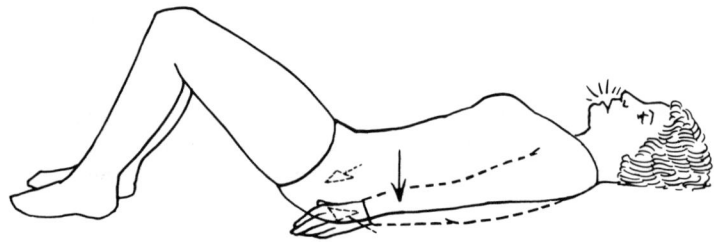

Repeat _____ times.

AS3 ABDOMINAL STRENGTHENING - STANDING

Bend your knees slightly, reach down and rest your hands on your thighs. Pull in your stomach while counting out loud to _____. Let go.

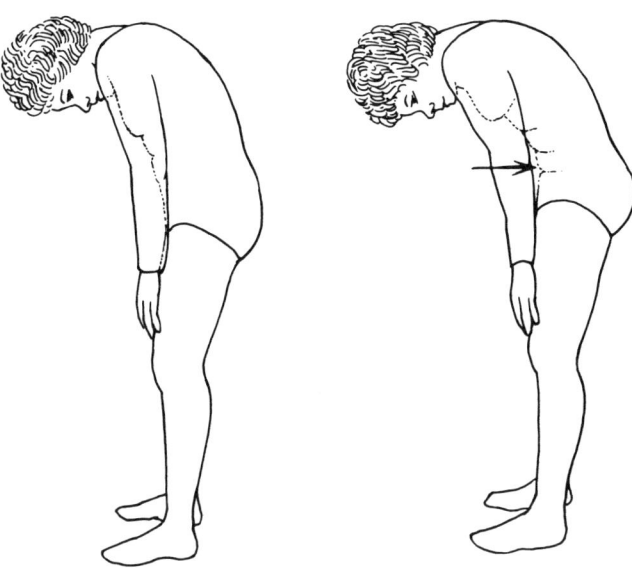

Repeat _____ times.

AS4 ABDOMINAL STRENGTHENING - ON HANDS AND KNEES

Assume a hands-and-knees position, with your hands underneath your shoulders, and knees shoulder-width apart. Do not bend your elbows throughout the entire exercise.

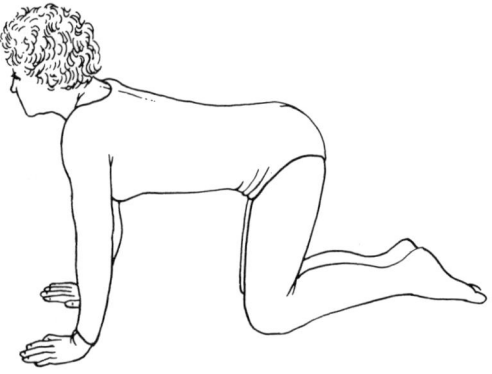

Drop your head, pull in your stomach muscles, and try to get your back as round and as high as possible. Exhale while assuming this position to the count of _____. Inhale as you raise your head up and return to starting position. Hold for a count of _____.

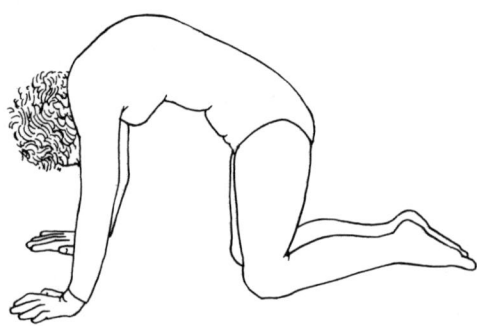

Repeat this entire exercise _____ times.

A Complete Low-Back Exercise Program

AS5 ABDOMINAL STRENGTHENING - BACK-LYING

Lie on your back with one pillow under knees, and your arms at your side.

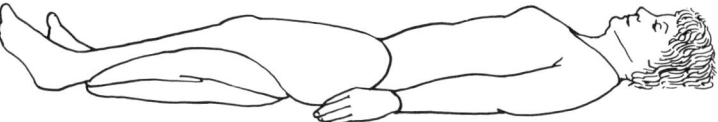

Begin to exhale slowly while you lift your head. Lift up only far enough so that you can see your navel. Exhale by counting out loud to six. Return to the floor, gently roll your head from side to side.

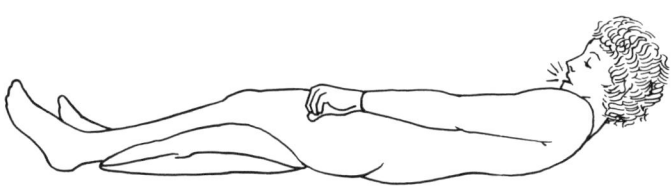

Inhale and prepare to repeat _____ times.

AS6 ABDOMINAL STRENGTHENING - BACK-LYING

Lie on your back with one pillow under your knees and your arms at your side.

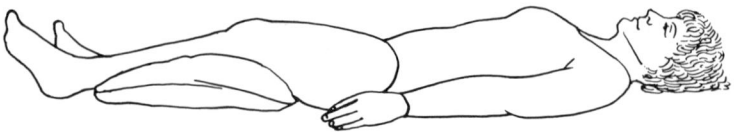

Exhale slowly by counting to three while you curl up beginning with your head until shoulder blades are off the floor. Hold here and finish counting to six. Slowly return to floor by uncurling with head reaching floor last. Roll head from side to side.

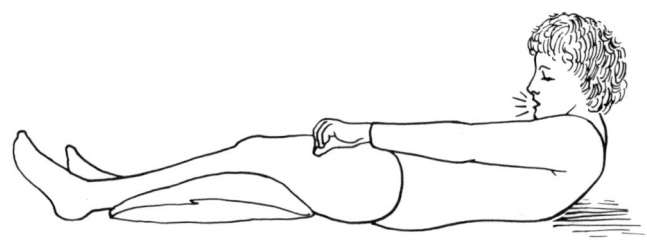

Inhale and repeat _____ times.

AS7 ABDOMINAL STRENGTHENING - BACK-LYING

Lie on your back, with feet flat on the floor and both knees bent. Keep arms at sides.

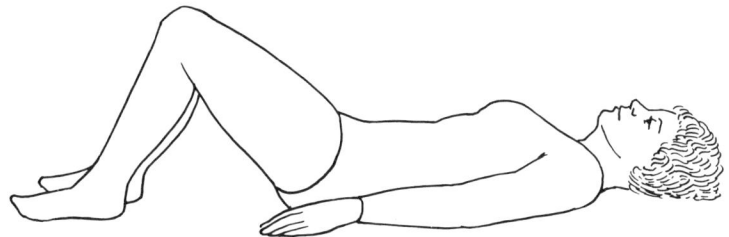

Bring left knee up toward your chest. Begin to exhale slowly by counting to three as you lift your head, and try to touch your forehead to your left knee. Hold this position and finish count to six.

Return head and foot to floor and roll your head gently from side to side. Inhale and prepare to repeat with the right leg.

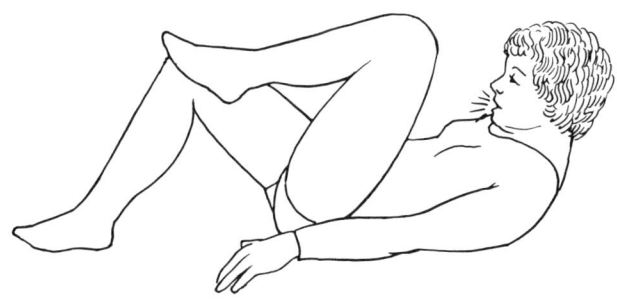

Repeat _____ times with each leg.

AS8 ABDOMINAL STRENGTHENING - BACK-LYING

Lie on your back with knees bent and feet flat on floor.

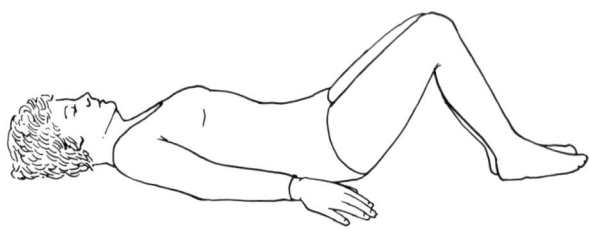

Bring both knees simultaneously to chest. Exhale and lift your head trying to touch your forehead to your knees while counting out loud to six.

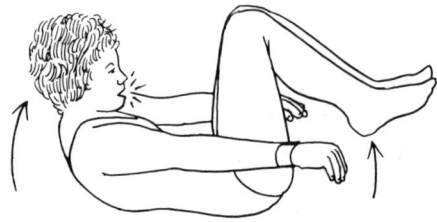

Return head and then legs to floor. Roll your head gently from side to side.

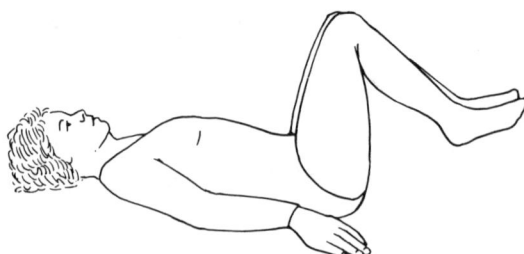

Inhale and repeat _____ times.

AS9 ABDOMINAL STRENGTHENING - BACK-LYING

Lie on your back with knees bent and feet flat on floor.

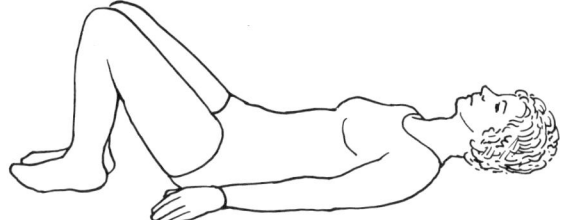

Lift your right knee up toward your chest to the count of six.

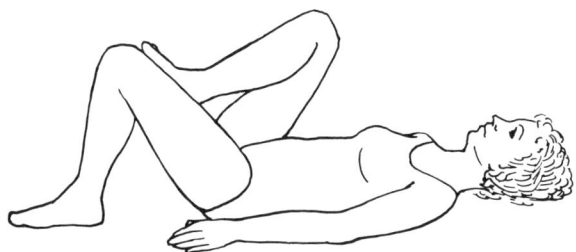

Tuck your chin, begin to exhale and then lift your left shoulder off the floor toward your right knee. Your arms are reaching toward the right knee. Return your left shoulder, head and then right foot to the floor. Roll your head from side to side. Inhale and repeat with left knee to right shoulder.

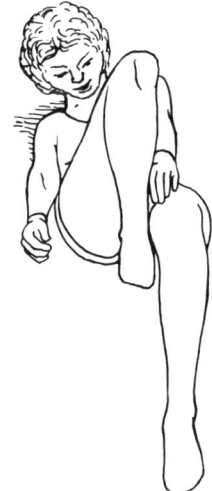

Repeat _____ times to each side.

AS10 ABDOMINAL STRENGTHENING - BACK-LYING

Lie on your back with knees bent and feet flat on floor.

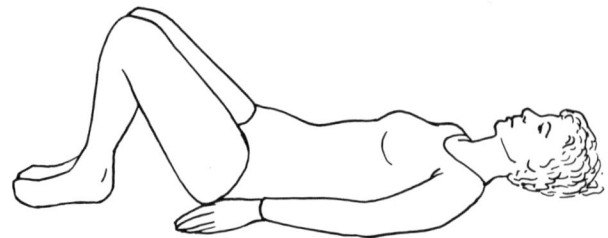

Tuck chin on chest and to the count of six curl up, bringing left shoulder toward right knee. Arms should be reaching forward toward right knee.

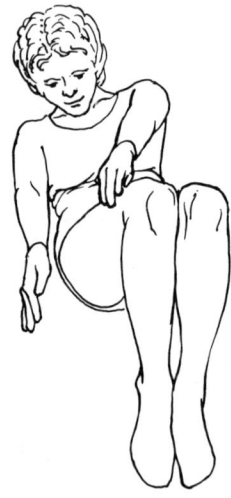

Return your left shoulder and head to the floor. Roll your head from side to side. Inhale and repeat with right shoulder toward left knee.

Repeat_____times to each side.

A Complete Low-Back Exercise Program

BES1 LOW BACK STRENGTHENING - STOMACH-LYING

Place two or three pillows under your stomach, keeping your hands at your side.

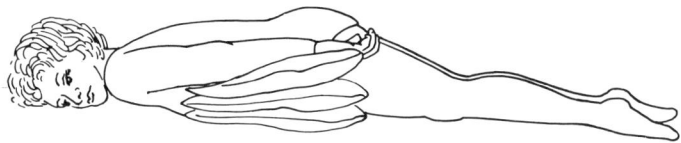

Keeping the knee straight, lift one leg off the floor until it is even with the level of the pillows. Hold and count out loud to six. Return the leg to the floor and roll it from side to side. Alternate legs.

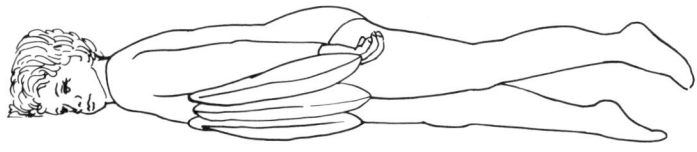

Repeat _____ times with each leg.

BES2 LOW BACK STRENGTHENING - STOMACH-LYING

Place two or three pillows under your stomach. Grasp a heavy piece of furniture for stabilization.

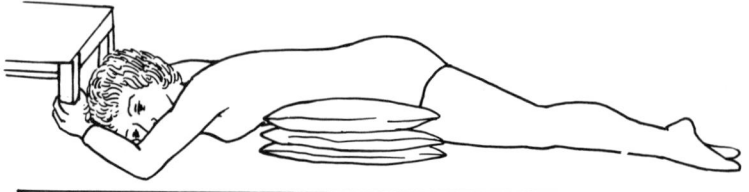

Keep your knees straight and lift both legs simultaneously off the floor until they are level with the pillows. Hold and count out loud to six. Return your legs to the floor and roll them from side to side.

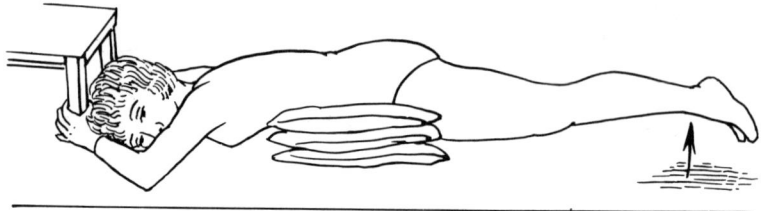

Repeat _____ times.

BES3 UPPER BACK STRENGTHENING - STOMACH-LYING

Place two or three pillows under your abdomen, and place your arms at your side (hands behind neck). Put feet under a heavy piece of furniture for stabilization.

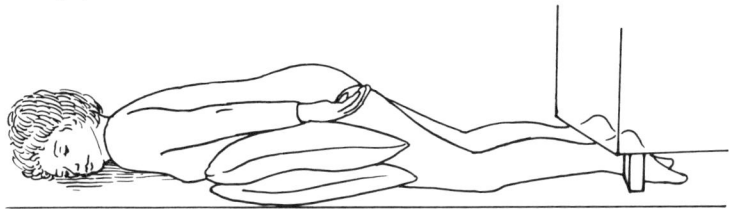

While exhaling, raise your head and chest off the floor. Raise up only to the point where your body will be even with the level of the pillows. Do not arch your back. Hold this position and count out loud to six. Return to the floor and let go completely.

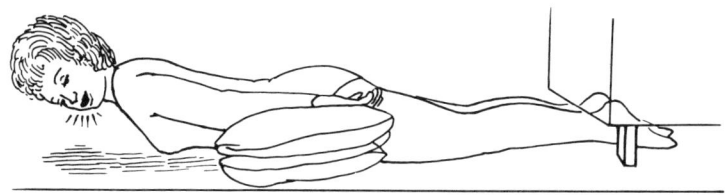

Repeat_____times.

BES4 BACK STRENGTHENING - STOMACH-LYING

Place two or three pillows under your stomach. Extend left arm straight forward over your head. Simultaneously lift left arm and right leg with knee straight until they are level with the pillow. Hold for the count of six. Let go. Repeat with right arm and left leg.

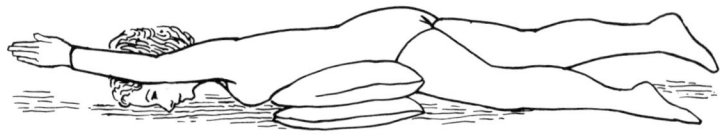

Repeat_____times with each side.

A Complete Low-Back Exercise Program

TFL1 STRETCH FOR THE TENSOR FASCIAE LATAE - BACK-LYING

Lie on your back, with your knees bent and feet flat on the floor.

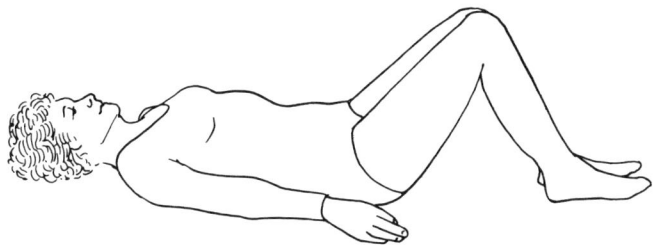

Gently drop both knees to the right, and let them rest completely on the floor for 15 seconds. You should use no effort to hold them there.

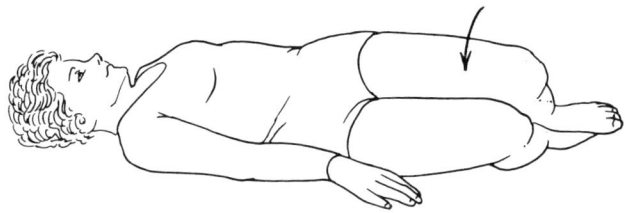

Return to the starting position and drop to the left.

Repeat _____ times to each side.

TFL2 STRETCH FOR THE TENSOR FASCIAE LATAE - SIDE-LYING

Lie on your right side. Keep bottom leg bent and extend left knee and hip so that left leg is behind right. Hold for 15 seconds. Then relax and bend left leg.

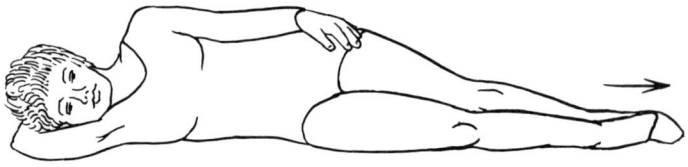

Turn on left side and repeat with right leg.

Repeat _____ times with each leg.

TFL3 STRETCH FOR THE TENSOR FASCIAE LATAE - SIDE-LYING

Lie on your side on the edge of the bed, facing the middle of the bed. Bend bottom leg up close to chest.

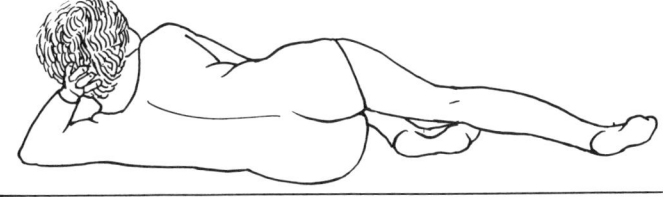

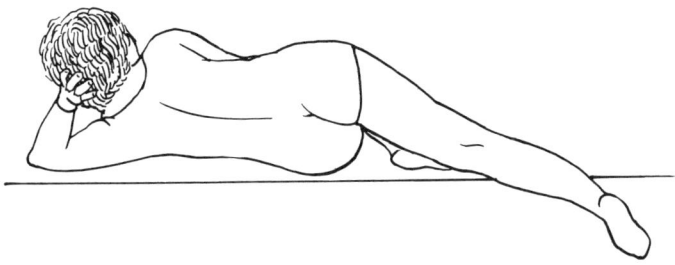

Keep top leg straight at hip and knee. Bring it back behind bottom leg, and allow it to dangle over the edge of the bed. Do not arch back. Hold for 15 seconds. Bend leg and return it to the bed.

Repeat with other leg.

Repeat _____ times with each leg.

HAdS1 HIP ADDUCTOR STRETCHING - BACK-LYING

Lie on your back with knees bent and feet flat on floor.

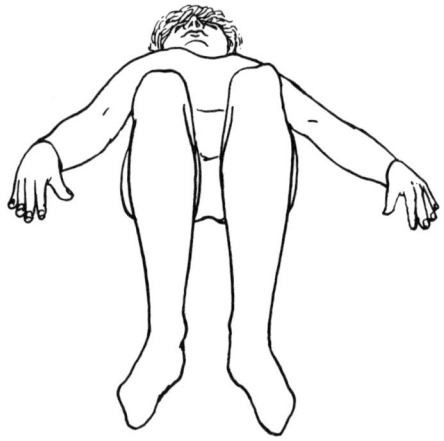

Hook right foot behind left heel. Let the right leg fall gently to the right. Hold there for 15 seconds. Return to starting position and repeat with left leg.

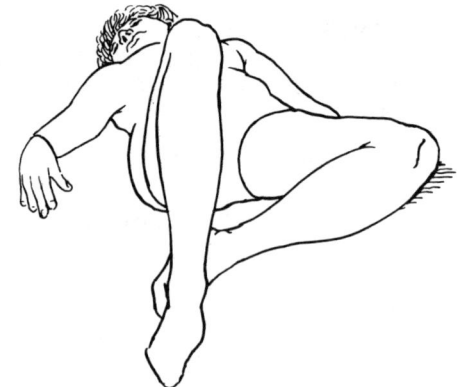

Repeat _____ times on each side.

HAdS2 HIP ADDUCTOR STRETCHING - SITTING

Sit on the floor, with your legs outstretched in a "v" position. Bend your knees so that you can bring the soles of your feet together with your hands.

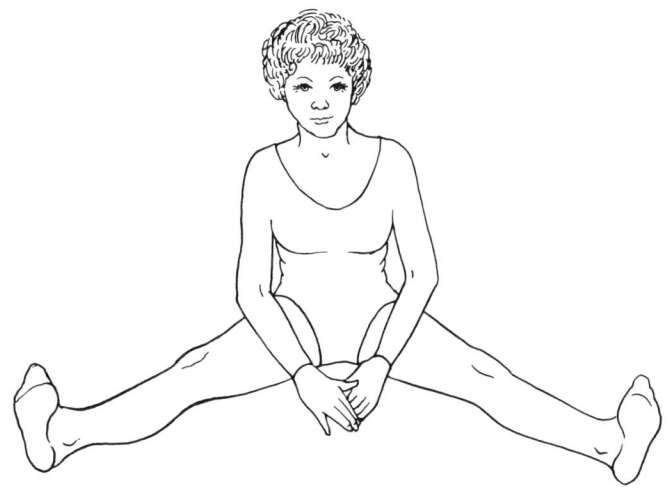

Continue to hold onto the top part of your feet with your hands, and bend over slightly so that your elbows rest on your inner knee. Gently press down with your elbows in an attempt to lower your knees to the floor.

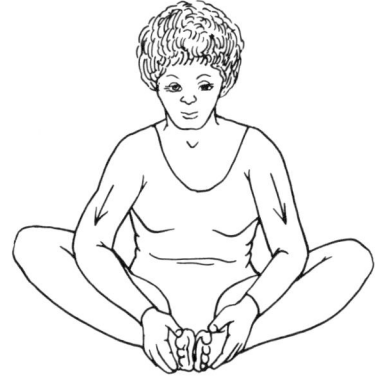

Hold the press for as long as is comfortable, up to 15 seconds. Do not bounce, or force the movement. You should feel the "pull" on both inner thighs. Release your hold.

Repeat _____ times.

SUMMARY

Theoretically, this program consists of treatment of muscle spasm, postinjection therapy, along with relaxation, limbering, flexibility, and strengthening components. As with any professional physical therapy plan, both short- and long-term goals, together with constant reevaluation procedures, are required, as is deemed necessary for the effective progression of the patient's treatment.

This will be discussed in detail in Chap. 5, along with ADL performance and functional carryover into the patient's lifestyle.

Chapter 5

Treatment/Management of the Low-Back Patient

INTRODUCTION

Now that you have the history of the patient, the results of the complete patient assessment, and the components of an effective "low-back program," you are ready to construct an effective, individualized treatment program for your patient. Here are some principles to remember throughout this chapter:

1. Always construct a program to fit your patient; do not try to fit the patient into a program.
2. Patient education should be utmost in your mind, and is always an important short-term goal of the therapist. It makes the long-term goal of discharging a patient who is functional, because he is knowledgable enough to apply the components of his program correctly to his individual situation, a reality.
3. Effective motivation is important in this program, and more so with back patients in general, because they must continue on an independent exercise program indefinitely to prevent further episodes.
4. The patient must understand the concepts of the treatment program, and his own back problem, so that eventually his exercise program will become an adjunct to other activities in his life, rather than a hindrance in preventing him from returning to a functional and enjoyable lifestyle of his choice.
5. The program of treatment must be well structured to be effective, yet, it must be flexible enough to allow for day-to-day changes in the condition of the patient.

6. The therapist must continually reevaluate the patient's condition.
7. The program must be progressive, and either be continually advanced or regressed, to match the condition of the patient at any given time.
8. Both the therapist and the patient must always have, and clearly understand, their respective goals within the program.
9. The patient must be taught to differentiate between pain and discomfort.
10. The therapist must keep in close communication with the physician.

With these principles in mind, the therapist is able to logically establish an effective treatment plan for the patient from either the physician's prescription or from the results of the patient-assessment worksheet or both.

TREATMENT COMPONENT VS. PATIENT SYMPTOMS

Table 1 represents the low-back pathologies that will be seen by the therapist most often. Note that the clinical manifestations between classifications differ much more than the symptoms to be treated by the therapist. This reinforces the fact that the symptoms being treated might be similar from patient to patient, but that the etiology of pain and source of the primary pathology differ substantially and should be of ongoing concern to the therapist/physician. Once the symptoms of pain, muscle spasm, etc., are reduced, the goal of the treatment should be to reduce the effects of the primary pathology. Therefore, treatment should not end when the symptoms have subsided, but when the underlying cause of the symptoms has been identified and treated. In this manner, the patient can be discharged with a complete physical therapy program for maintenance of symptoms (ice, limbering, relaxation) should an exacerbation occur and for improvement of muscle strength, flexibility, and function, in addition to medication, injections, curtailment of activities, bracing, and supports for the more serious skeletal etiologies as described by the physician. This total approach to the treatment and management of patients has proven very successful at New York Hospital where the majority of patients (without severe psychological manifestations) return to a functional and enjoyable lifestyle.

Table 1

Etiology of Primary pathology	Primary pathology	Clinical manifestations	Typical presenting symptoms to be treated by the therapist
Degenerative disease Trauma	Facet dysfunction Vertebral instability Nerve Root tension, irritation, compression. Ligament sprains	Pain (can be radiating and/or referred), loss of motion, instability, neurological signs, condition aggravated by activity, reduced by rest. Patient will usually lie still by choice. Usually presents with negative roentgenogram.	Pain, muscle spasm, loss of motion and mobility, instability, loss of muscle strength, loss of flexibility, increased muscle tension, loss of functional capabilities, loss of normal movement.
Congenital and acquired skeletal anomalies	Facet dysfunction Spondlyolisthesis Scoliosis Increased lumbar lordosis Compression fracture Osteoporosis Osteoarthritis Laminectomies Fusion	Pain (intermittent), exaggerated by an increase in activity. Some loss of mobility, structural changes present, positive roentgenograms, usually no neurological signs.	Pain, muscle spasm, increase in muscle tension, loss of mobility, loss of flexibility, loss of functional capabilities, loss of normal movement.
Acquired muscular pathology	Increased tension Triggerpoint Strain Muscle imbalance Contracture Muscle spasm Muscle weakness Trauma Fibrositis Tendonitis	Pain, loss of mobility, stiffness with rest, activity is aggravating. Usually no neurological signs.	Pain increase in muscle tension, muscle spasm, loss of flexibility, loss of muscle strength, loss of functional capabilities.
Systemic Disease	To be treated by the physician		

Here are the Treatment Components, most of which are described in Chap. 4, from which the therapist will form the treatment program:

  Patient education
  Relaxation training
  Limbering
  Flexibility exercises
  Muscle strengthening exercises
  ADL training
  Transcutaneous nerve stimulator
  Bracing and supports
  Other modalities
    Ice or ethyl chloride
    Heat
    Massage
    Electric stimulation
    Ultrasound
    Mobilization
  Maintenance-oriented program
  Functional program
  (Drugs and injections by the physician)

As reflected by Table 1, here is a list of the most common symptoms and conditions that the therapist will treat with the above components:

  Pain
  Muscle spasm
  Increased muscle tension
  Lack of flexibility
  Muscle weakness
  Muscle inbalance
  Limited ROM
  Contracture
  Triggerpoints
  Ligamentous sprain
  Muscle strain
  Skeletal strain
  Fibrositis
  Abnormal gait
  Loss of normal movement (specific and/or gross)
  Loss of functional capacity
  Improper body mechanics

DIFFERENTIATION OF TREATMENT

Although there are no clear-cut categories of treatment procedures, the following differentiations are presented to orient the therapist in recognizing several levels of treatment. The level of treatment will usually be established by the physician's diagnosis and/or the therapist's interpretation of the patient-assessment worksheet.

The Treatment Components are not in any particular order, and the listing should not represent their priority in treatment, or, correspondence to any symptom in the column on the left.

Treatment of Acute Episode

Most Common Presenting Symptoms/Conditions	Treatment Components
Pain	Patient education
Spasm	Modalities
Increased muscle tension	Limbering
Ligament strain	ADL during the acute stage
Muscle strain	Bracing and supports
Skeletal sprain and/or instability	Injection and postinjection treatments avoidance of aggravating movements
Triggerpoints	

Maintenance-Oriented Treatment Program

Most Common Presenting Symptoms/Conditions	Treatment Components
Pain	Patient education
Increased muscle tension	Relaxation training
Lack of flexibility	Modalities
Muscle weakness	Limbering exercises
Muscle imbalance	Flexibility exercises
Contracture	Muscle strengthening exercises
Triggerpoint	ADL training
Fibrositis	Bracing and supports
Skeletal strain and/or instability	Postinjection treatments
Loss of normal movement (specific) and/or gross)	Mobilization
Body mechanics	

Functional Program

Most Common Presenting Symptoms/Conditions	Treatment Components
Increased muscle tension	Patient Education
Loss of normal movement (neuromuscular coordination)	Reevaluation (with specificity)
	Specificity of Exercise
Improper body mechanics	Proper body mechanics

Of course, the Treatment Components presented are not the only ones available to apply to the Presenting Symptoms/Conditions, but they are methods that are most effective. If several combinations of components are not successful, the therapist should report this to the physician, and together, they will establish new treatment guidelines.

APPLICATION OF THE LOW-BACK EXERCISE PROGRAM

Patient #1

The patient-assessment sheet on page 139 represents a typical low-back patient that you as a therapist are confronted with daily. Traditionally, she would probably receive a hot pack and five or six exercises and be on her way. Both the therapist and the patient would be confused as to why an exacerbation of symptoms occur, or why the patient fails to respond to treatment. Let's examine the patient's condition to explain this response of failure to traditional treatment.

The first step is, of course, to list the patient's symptoms/conditions. This is done for you by surveying the Pain Assessment (2) sheet. The results are listed as

Increased muscle tension	Lack of flexibility
Muscle weakness	Loss of normal movement
Pain	Loss of functional capacity
Triggerpoint	Improper body mechanics
Spasm	

The second is to identify which symptoms are to be treated, and in what order; pain is always the first consideration. In this case the spasm and triggerpoint are most likely at the root of the patient's immediate pain. Since the triggerpoint cannot be injected while the

Name __PATIENT #1__ Age __40__
History no. __10354b__ Dx __MUSCLE SPASM__
Date __10/1__ Examiner __JGL__

Pain Assessment (2)

Where is the Pain?

As INDICATED

10/1

K-W TEST
Abd - 2
HF - 10
Abd+HF - 9
UBE - 5
LBE - 10

11/2

K-W TEST
Add - 9
HF - 10
Abd+HF - 9
UBE - 10
LBE - 10

Shade in painful area:
- ↑↓ rotation R or L
- = spasm
- ∨ stiff segment
- ⊗ triggerpoint
- ∭ fibrositis

Annotations on body diagram:
- INCREASED MUSCLE TENSION
- muscle WEAKNESS
- PAIN
- LACK OF FLEXIBILITY

Loss of normal movement
Loss of functional capacity
Improper body mechanics

muscle is in spasm, treatment to break the cycle of the painful contraction should begin immediately. It is specifically detailed in Chap. 4. The patient's follow-up treatment at home with ice treatment and relaxation and gentle limbering must augment the physical therapist's efforts, since the muscle in spasm must be kept at its resting length for several days before the spasm will be sufficiently interrupted. At this point the therapist should introduce exercise LBS6, to be preceded by electric stimulation, ice, relaxation, and limbering, to allow the muscle sufficient range to contract normally without returning to the "spasm" state.

Usually 2 to 3 days of this treatment is sufficient to break a muscle spasm and return the muscle to its resting state along with normal gentle contractions of the muscle. However, if the spasm is stubborn and will not respond to this treatment or if it does respond but immediately returns to the spasm state, the therapist must entertain two considerations: one is that the treatment is not frequent enough or is not being done correctly, or, secondly, that a more serious pathology (i.e., vertebral instability, nerve root compression) may be the underlying etiology of pain.

During the time the patient is being treated for an acute muscle spasm, it is best to use large ice packs or plastic bags of ice cubes for 30 minutes over the painful area to produce the desired anesthetic result. If the patient is in agonizing pain, the ice treatment should precede electric stimulation so the added stimuli will not reinforce the spasm. The first 10 minutes of the electrotherapy should be of a tetanizing current, and at a very low setting, dependent on the patient's tolerance. If the current is too strong, it, too may reinforce the spasm. Ten minutes of alternating current should follow the tetanizing current to induce gentle, normal contractions of the painful muscle.

This treatment is followed by the breathing, relaxation, and limbering exercises. Should the patient feel pain during the limbering exercises, the therapist may either return the ice pack for 5 to 10 minutes or spray the area with ethyl chloride as the patient exercises. However, special care must be taken if the area has previously been frozen. The appearance of a white residue or an extreme burning sensation reported by the patient are contraindications for further cold application. The patient must not feel pain while exercising, as the painful stimuli may cause an exacerbation of the spasm.

Assuming that the patient is now free of the painful spasm, the patient assessment is presently completed. It may be at this point that the triggerpoint is first identified (or in the initial examination if the spasm was not in effect at that time) and the remaining symptoms/conditions listed above will be uncovered. At this point the physician may wish to inject the triggerpoint if it is painful to the patient and if the physician feels it is the etiology of the patient's painful state. If this is the case, three postinjection treatments listed in detail in Chap. 4 will follow the injection.

If the patient experiences muscle spasm, hematoma, or pain after the injection by the physician, an ice pack should be used as part of the follow-up treatment. Otherwise, ethyl chloride spray is sufficient. Fifteen minutes of surging current is followed by relaxation and limbering exercises. The patient should also receive a full explanation of theory and review of all written material that is given to him at that time. Instructions in home treatment and ADL activities should also be provided. The therapist should be aware of the fact that the patient must be kept in an active role whenever possible. The patient is responsible for follow-up treatments at home, for icing when pain is present, for exercising, and for the application of proper body positioning during daily activities. This concept benefits the patient in two ways: he or she has the option of chosing his or her degree of responsibility to the program and, thus, its success, and this participation allows the patient the opportunity to exercise control over his or her pain and disability to a great degree. The patient deserves this type of involvement in his or her treatment program.

After the third treatment, if any other triggerpoints are present, the physician would find this the most appropriate time to inject them. Of course, they would be followed by an additional three posttriggerpoint injection treatments by the therapist. Assuming, now, that the patient received relief from the primary pain resulting from the muscle spasm, and had favorable results from treatment of the triggerpoint, it is the proper time to consider the other symptoms/conditions listed on the Pain Assessment Sheet.

It is important to consider muscle flexibility before strengthening exercises are prescribed. A shortened muscle will often go into spasm or the individual muscle fibers will tear and form additional triggerpoints should the muscle be stretched too vigorously from a shortened position caused by disuse or repeated contractions. Therefore, flexibility exercises should be added gradually and in progression until the patient reaches within 10 to 15% normal flexibility before strengthening exercises are included in the treatment program.

At this point it is important to help patients in differentiating between discomfort and pain. Hamstring stretching is ideal for this. Patients are asked to pay special attention to the "feeling" that accompanies hamstring stretching. Do they interpret this as pain? Is it the same feeling they have during an episode of back pain. If so, then it is not pain at all that they feel in their backs, but rather, abnormal muscles trying to work in a normal manner. Many times patients will complain that they cannot perform their exercises because of pain, and on questioning them, it is this same "discomfort" of muscle stretching that they feel, and not pain. Patients should expect to feel some discomfort while exercising, but not pain. Exercises that cause true intensification of pain should be temporarily eliminated from the treatment program.

The most important exercises to include for this patient in terms of flexibility would be Low Back Extensor Stretching (with and without rotation) and Hamstring Stretching. In terms of muscle strengthening the Kraus-Weber test reveals weakness in the abdominals and upper back extensors. In addition, once proper flexibility has been regained in the lower back, stregthening of the lower back extensors should always be included.

By this time the patient should have begun to regain normal movement because the pian has been eliminated, and flexibility and muscle strength have been improved. Next, the patient is taught to incorporate these normal movements together with proper body mechanics (as described in Chap. 6) as prevention against further injury, and in preparation for further conditioning for sports or other recreational activities.

Here is the patient's treatment program:

Presenting Symptom/Condition   Treatment Component Used

Treatment of the Actute Episode

Dx: Muscle spasm   Rx: Modalities
                                    Ice
                                    Electric stimulation
                                  Relaxation training
                                  Limbering exercises
                                  Patient education
                                    Home program
                                  Reevaluation

Goal: To reduce pain and muscle spasm

Treatment/Management of the Low-Back Patient

Dx: Triggerpoint

Rx: Postinjection treatment
Modalities
   Ice/ethyl chloride
   Electric stimulation
Relaxation training
Limbering exercises
Patient education
   Home program
Reevaluation

Goal: To reduce effects of triggerpoint

Maintenance-Oriented Program

Dx: Increased muscle tension
Decreased flexibility
Decreased muscle strength
Loss of normal movement
Loss of functional capacity
Improper body mechanics

Rx: Modalities
Relaxation training
Flexibility exercises
Strengthening exercises
ADL activities
Proper body mechanics
Patient education
   Home program
Reevaluation

Since this patient did not wish to return to any athletic or recreational activity, she did not require a functional program to prepare her for any specific activity. Her long-term goal, therefore, was to return to activities of daily living with normal movement and no pain.

Here is this patient's treatment program:

Patients Name: PATIENT #1
Hosp. #: 103546
Inpatient PA OPD PHS.Comp.:
MD Name:
P.T. Name: J.G.L.
Date of 1st Tx.: 10/1

#	R	L	P	LBS	HAS	HES	HS	HFS	AS	BES	TFL	HAdS
1	10/1	10/1										
2	10/1	10/1					10/7		10/12	10/20		
3	10/1	10/1					10/9			10/15		
4				10/7			10/10		10/12			
5				10/9								
6				10/3								
7				10/10					10/14			
8												
9									10/14			
10									10/15			

N.Y.H. 99319

When exercise is taught to patient, date and initial appropriate box above.
Date and initial below when sheet given to patient:
  –How to perform the exercises 10/1   –Your home treatment 10/1
  –Questions and answers 10/1   –General relaxation 10/1

(COMMENTS ON REVERSE)

You can see from this case presentation that the traditional hot pack and five or six standard exercises could not possibly treat the patient's muscle spasm, triggerpoint, and other specific conditions with any degree of competence. In fact, it may have made conditions worse. It is imperative that each patient be considered an individual entity by the therapist, and that the therapist logically establish a treatment program that corresponds to the patient's symptoms.

Patient #2

Patient #2 presents with an anterior pelvic tilt, resulting in an increased lordosis, but with negative roentgenograms. Tight hip flexors and rectus femoris bilaterally, along with lack of muscle strength in the hamstrings and tightness in the paraspinal muscles of the back, are usually responsible for this condition. The patient complains of pain across the low back when standing and sitting for prolonged periods, and since he is a draftsman, it is especially disabling. The Kraus-Weber test confirms the muscular picture of an anterior pelvic tilt: weak abdominals; strong hip flexors, which lack flexibility and pull the vertebra forward causing pain and increased lordosis; and weak low-back and hamstring muscles.

Here is the patient's treatment program:

Presenting Symptom/Condition   Treatment Components Used

Treatment of the Acute Episode

No muscle spasm present
No triggerpoint present   None

Maintenance-Oriented Program

Dx: Increased muscle tension   Rx: Modalities
     Decreased flexibility   Relaxation training
     Decreased muscle strength   Flexibility exercises
     Pain with normal movements   Strengthening exercises
       and posture   Proper body mechanics
     Improper body mechanics   Patient education
                                            Home program
                                      Reevaluation

Goal: To return the patient to pain-free status during normal movements and posture, especially standing and sitting

Name PATIENT #2
History no. 123456
Date 2/20

Age 26
Dx MUSCLE IMBALANCE
Examiner JGL

Pain Assesment (2)

Where is the Pain?
Across low back

2/20	4/15
K-W TEST	K-W
Abd -2	10
HF -10 ē PAIN 10	
Add+HF -3 ē PAIN 10	
UBE -10	10
LBE -4	10

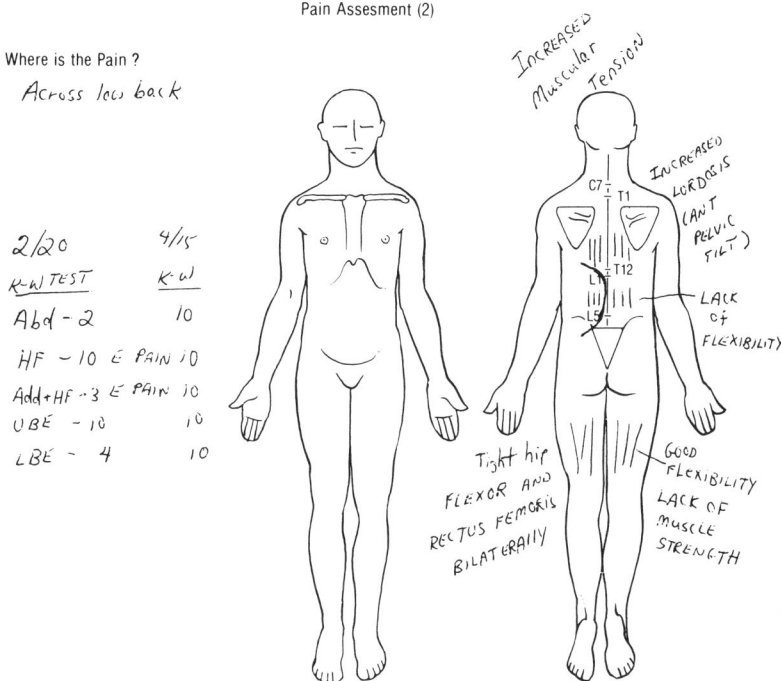

INCREASED Muscular Tension
INCREASED LORDOSIS (ANT PELVIC TILT)
LACK of FLEXIBILITY
Tight hip FLEXOR AND RECTUS FEMORIS BILATERALLY
GOOD FLEXIBILITY LACK OF MUSCLE STRENGTH

Pain with normal movements
Improper body mechanics

Shade in painful area:
↻↺ rotation R or L
= spasm
V stiff segment
⊗ triggerpoint
≀≀≀ fibrositis

Here is his maintanence program:

Patients Name	Hosp. #	Inpatient PA OPD PHS.Comp.	MD Name	P.T. Name	Date of 1st Tx.
PATIENT #2	453116			J.G.L.	2/20

#	R	L	P	LBS	HAS	HES	HS	HFS	AS	BES	TFL	HAdS
1	2/20	2/20	2/20				PRE's AND MANUAL RESISTANCE TO HAMSTRINGS	2/20				
2	2/20	2/20	2/24					2/24		3/6		
3	2/20	2/20	3/2									
4			3/5	3/2				3/1	2/20			
5												
6				2/20					2/20			
7									2/26			
8									3/1			
9									3/5			
10									3/6			

N.Y.H. .When exercise is taught to patient, date and initial appropriate box above.
.Date and initial below when sheet given to patient:
99319 –How to perform the exercises 2/26 –Your home treatment 2/26 (COMMENTS
–Questions and answers 2/20 –General relaxation 2/20 ON REVERSE)

This program consists of relaxation, limbering, pelvic tilting, low-back stretching, hip flexor stretching, abdominal strengthening, and back extensor strengthening. Manual resistance and PRE's are prescribed for strengthening of the hamstrings. One of two exercises can be added at each therapy appointment. When one exercise becomes too "easy" for the patient to perform, i.e., he does not feel any results from the movement, then it should be eliminated from the program, and a progression substituted.

Fifteen minutes of surging current, with two electrodes on each side of the low back, would be an appropriate modality. Ethyl chloride spray when and if needed during the exercise program for the paraspinal muscles would also be indicated. Most important with Patient #2 would be that he learn an awareness of the "tilt" of the pelvis and that he be encouraged to maintain the tilt during ADL activities, especially sitting and standing. This must be done gradually, however, otherwise muscle strain may occur. The patient can be informed about performing the pelvic tilt in elevators, buses, subways, the office, etc., while leaning against any available wall or solid area. The therapist must make the patient's life easier and more enjoyable by adding components to the patient's program that can be performed during a routine day in his life. Methods that complicate or take up too much time are usually discarded by the patient, and are replaced by old habits.

Patient #2 made good progress and was able to return to work with an exercise program suited to his job requirements. He relearned how to sit correctly, to perform LBS6 and get up and walk after sitting for a prolonged period. He kept his feet on a stool so that his knees were higher than his hips to reduce the pull of the hips flexons, and he was encouraged to buy the proper chair with a back support and arm rests. He continued on his maintenance program and needed no follow-up treatment.

Patient #3

Initially, Patient #3 was transported to the Physical Therapy Department on a stretcher. He could not roll, sit, bend or raise his left leg without excruciating pain. Prior to the first physical therapy treatment he had been in the hospital as an in-patient for a period of four days undergoing intensive diagnostic testing, i.e., roentgenogram, myelogram, EMG, all of which were negative. The patient was 6'4" tall, slim, and 29 years old.

The physician's original diagnosis was that of possible herniated nucleus pulposus (HNP) with root compression at L_4, L_5, S_1, with the most immediate symptom being muscle spasm. Therefore, the patient received the treatment previously described, both to eliminate pain from the spasm and to allow a more complete assessment. Before treatment could begin, however, the first problem of the therapist was to roll the patient over onto his stomach. Here is a procedure that works well: one pillow is placed across the patient's abdomen and another one between his knees. He is instructed to raise his arms overhead and roll his body "like a log" onto the pillow that is across his abdomen. If two therapists are available, one should stand behind the patient and help push him onto the pillow (with one hand on his shoulder and one on his pelvis) while the other therapist stands facing the patient and pulls him onto the pillow (by holding his uppermost arm and the top leg). The pillow is then removed from between the knees and placed at the bottom of the plinthe so the patient can rest his feet on it. This is the most mechanically correct prone position for the low-back patient.

Once the patient was properly positioned he received two large ice packs to the low-back area for 30 minutes, even though the spasm was palpable just on the left. Often the pain will radiate to the opposite side, or the patient will shift his weight to an unnatural position and cause spasm on the opposite side. Many times a patient will report, "When I went home my left side felt great and all the pain was gone, but soon after I had the same pain on the right side." Treating both sides with ice and electric stimulation will often prevent this.

Name **PATIENT #3**   Age **29**
History no. **143765**   Dx **POSSIBLE HNP with RT COMPRESSION**
Date **8/19**   Examiner **JGL**

Pain Assesment (2)

Where is the Pain?

INITIALLY. ACROSS LBE RADIATION
INTO (L) LEG..
AFTER SPASM WAS RELIEVED;
PAIN LOCALIZED IN (L)
BUTTOCKS AT ILIAC
CREST & SOME
RADIATION

K-W TEST
ABD - 7
HF 2 pain
ABD + HF - 4 pain
UBE - 3 pain
LBE - 9

UNEQUAL LEG LENGTH L < R
ROM of (L) HIP : 90° & PAIN
SLR ON (L) = 30° & PAIN
NEG MYELOGRAM + X RAYS
NORMAL EMG; DTR's PRESENT

Shade in painful area:
↑↓ rotation R or L
= spasm
∀ stiff segment
⊗ triggerpoint
§ fibrositis

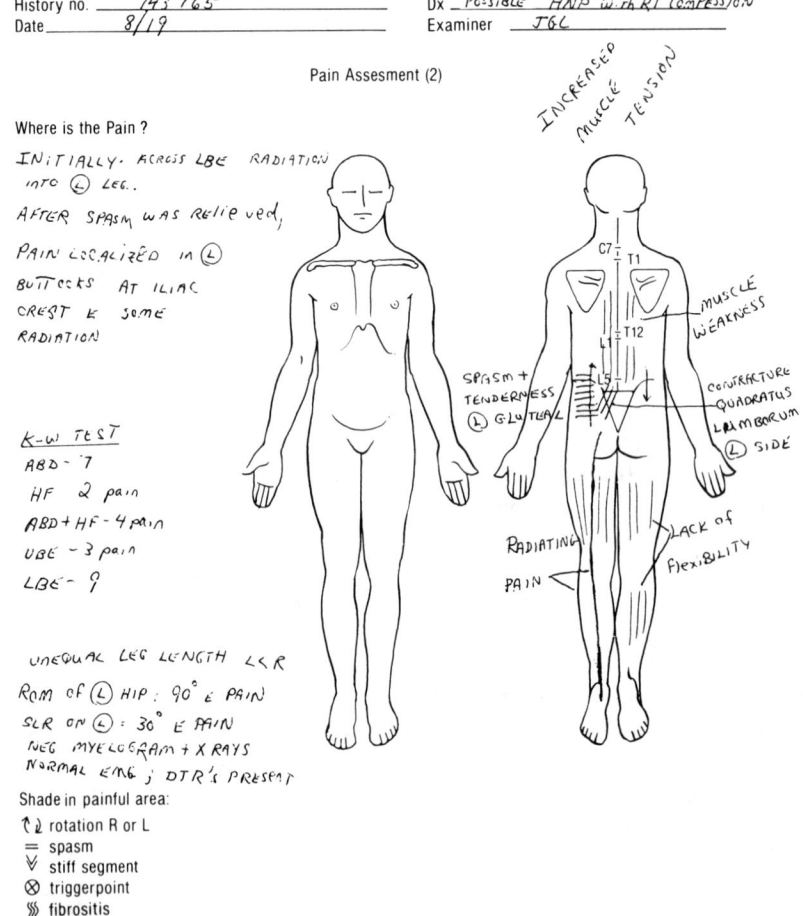

The patient received this treatment two times a day, and used ice in between times while he was in his hospital bed. He also practiced breathing, relaxation, and limbering exercises (even though he could not perform them through the range initially). In four days enough of the pain had subsided so that he could sit and roll over into the prone position independently. At this time the patient assessment was completed. Here are the results:

Pain
    left buttock at iliac crest
    left groin
    along sciatica
    lateral aspect of knee to left heel
Increased tension
Limited range of motion
    hip flexion on left, limited to 90° with pain
Spasm
    hamstring on the left
    abnormal pulling at ischial tuberosity on left
Abnormal gait
    patient could not put heel of left foot to floor, leans to the left.
Triggerpoint
    at insertion of paraspinal muscle at left iliac crest
Muscle weakness
    all major postural groups
Unequal leg length
    left < than right
Unequal pelvic height
    left ↑ than right
Lack of flexibility
    hamstrings, right and left
    calf
    paraspinal
    hip flexor, left
Decreased SLR
    right = 60°
    left = 30° with pain
Decreased circumference
    left calf (slightly)

Since the patient's pain was still a major concern, this treatment program was again geared to eliminate or at least to decrease it. The physician injected the triggerpoint in the left buttock area, and while the patient received the usual three postinjection therapy sessions, ice packs were applied to the left hamstring in an attempt to break the spasm in that area. From the beginning the patient complained of "a pain" at the left ischial tuberosity, in the hamstring, and at the lateral aspect of the knee. This would be the first clue, along with a painful and limited SLR, of a spasm in the hamstring. A gentle hamstring stretch (HS2) was added to the patient's exercise program, which he performed with the assistance of a therapist within his pain limitations. This treatment continued until the patient could perform a hamstring stretch without pain (and without prior ice treatment) to the point of elevation that he had reached the day before with ice (three days). This meant that the spasm was no longer present and from that time on, the patient received hot packs to both hamstring areas, while he received electric stimulation to the back, in an attempt to increase the elasticity of the hamstrings while stretching.

By this time the patient had progressed to the point of good bed mobility, he could roll, turn from prone to supine and back, come to a sitting position, and sit with feet dangling off the plinthe for increasingly longer periods of time daily. He was ambulating in the therapeutic pool for short periods. SLR had increased to 70° on the right and 50° on the left with stretching discomfort only, and no pain. However, he was still being transported to and from physical therapy by stretcher because of his inability to sit for any length of time.

These were the remaining problems:

Pain
    along sciatica (reduced)
    lateral aspect of knee to left heel (reduced)
    when sitting
Abnormal gait
    patient still cannot put heel to the floor, continues to lean to left.
Muscle weakness
    all major postural groups
Unequal leg length
    left < than right
Unequal pelvic height
    left ↑ than right
Lack of flexibility
    hamstring, right and left
    calf
    paraspinal
    hip flexor, left

As the treatment progressed, the patient's pain decreased substantially. He commented that "tightness" was replacing the pain, and now before exercising he felt "tight," whereas after exercising he felt "loose." The emphasis of the current treatment program was put on relaxation and flexibility. The patient was young, impatient, and in a driving occupation. The competition at his job was fierce, and he often remarked that "it felt good to be away." He was often "tense" and "tight" in between treatments.

Contract-relax techniques were used to stretch the hamstrings, in addition to all of the hamstring stretches listed in Chap. 4. Calf stretching against the wall and on stairs, LBS 6, and others listed on the patient's card were added gradually.

Up to this time, it was not known why the discrepancy in leg length or pelvic height was present. The patient had no scoliosis or other mechanical abnormality other than his gait deviation, which had been acquired shortly before his entering the hospital. However, once the patient had begun his flexibility program, the therapist noticed that his left quadratus lumborum did not have the normal range of motion, and that the hip was continually in the "hiked" position. After questioning the patient, it was learned that a few years earlier he had been an oarsman in college for several years and had continually exercised only the left side of his body. In this case, the rowing caused him to push forcefully down with both feet while he turned to the left rear. In the completion of this move, the pelvis is continually elevated, and because of the speed involved, an almost constant contraction was maintained. Subsequently, he had developed a contracture of the quadratus lumborum. Of course, stretching exercises using weights and positioning were added to correct this.

When the patient had reached 70° bilaterally of hamstring flexibility, and nearly normal movement in LBS6 and HS4, muscle strengthening exercises were added one or two at a time. They are listed in detail on the patient's card.

Five weeks after his first physical therapy treatment, the patient had acceptable muscle strength and flexibility. He was due for discharge in a few days and asked whether or not he was ready for handball and swimming, the two activities he had decided to return to in order to "keep in shape." Because of his interest in participating in a sport, this patient had to be conditioned to a level higher than either of the two previous patients.

Patients Name			Hosp. #	Inpatient PA OPD PHS.Comp.		MD Name		P.T. Name	Date of 1st Tx.	
PATIENT #3			654321					J.G.L.	8/19	
#	R	L	P	LBS	HAS	HES	HS	HFS	AS	BES	TFL	HAdS
1	8/19	8/19	9/2	8/28				8/27		9/5	8/29	
2	8/19	8/19	9/7		9/3 with wt.	9/3	8/24			9/6		9/9
3	8/19	8/19	9/8	8/29			8/28	9/4		9/6	9/7	
4				8/30			8/30	9/9				
5				8/31			8/31					
6				8/27			9/1					
7				9/1			9/2					
8							9/8					
9												
10												

N.Y.H. .When exercise is taught to patient, date ~~and initial~~ appropriate box above.
         .Date ~~and initial~~ below when sheet given to patient:
99319   —How to perform the exercises 8/19   —Your home treatment 8/19   (COMMENTS
         —Questions and answers   8/19   —General relaxation 8/19   ON REVERSE)

Therefore, after another reevaluation concentrating on power, speed, endurance, and strength was performed, a functional program was constructed with the patient's individual needs in mind.

As a review here are the patient's treatment programs from the beginning:

Presenting Symptom/Condition   Treatment Components Used

Treatment of the Acute Episode

Dx: Muscle spasm   Rx: Modalities
                                        Ice
                                        Electric stimulation
                                      Relaxation training
                                      Limbering exercises
                                      Patient education
                                      Reevaluation

Goal: To reduce pain and muscle spasm

Dx: Triggerpoint   Rx: Postinjection treatment
                                      Modalities
                                        Ice/ethyl chloride
                                        Electric stimulation
                                      Relaxation training
                                      Limbering exercises
                                      Flexibility exercise (HS2)
                                      Patient education
                                      Reevaluation

Goal: To reduce effects of triggerpoint

Maintenance-Oriented Program

Dx: Increased muscle tension
Decreased flexibility
Decreased muscle strength
Contracture
Abnormal gait
Loss of normal movement
Loss of functional capacity
Improper body mechanics

Rx: Modalities
Relaxation training
Flexibility exercises
Strengthening exercises
ADL activities
Proper body mechanics
Patient education
Reevaluation

Goal: To prepare patient for normal activities

Functional Program

Dx: Increased muscle tension
Loss of normal movement
Decreased muscle strength with coordinated movements
Need for proper warm-up and cool-down
Improper body mechanics

Rx: Patient education
Reevaluation (with specificity)
Specificity of exercise
Proper body mechanics

Goal: To prepare patient for recreational activities

Toward the end of the patient's hospital stay, he was exercising an average of four hours a day. This time was divided between morning and afternoon treatments. The amount of work he expended is also reflected in the extensive functional program he performed daily, first on an out-patient basis, then at a gym near his home. Of course, not all patients have either the time or effort necessary to exercise four hours a day, but in this case he did because of his hospitalization. Progress is much more impressive when a patient who has extensive limitations can be treated as an in-patient, or for at least a two-hour period every day as an out-patient.

Once a patient reaches his functional program he need only be reminded of the sport or activity that he will soon be able to return to, for motivation. As a matter of fact, all of these functional exercises should be related as much as possible to the patient's sport. An example would be to have the patient duplicate his skill movements with the pulleys or extract any part of the skill movement and have the patient repeat it several times as an exercise.

In the earlier treatment programs, exercises should be related to ADL activities as much as possible. A patient who sits at a desk all day would appreciate very much the statement: "Learning to do the pelvic tilt first in the supine position and then in the chair will allow you to sit for longer periods at your desk without pain." Whereas, an older patient would accept this as the basis for learning and practicing hamstring stretches: "These exercises will help to eliminate some of the tightness and cramping in the back of your thigh, and will also make it easier for you to go up and down stairs." If a patient is asked to spend his time on performing exercises, the request must be backed by a legitimate answer to the question, "Why?"

Here is Patient #3's functional program:

Relaxation

Limbering

Flexibility
    one stretch per major muscle group (held for 15 to 30 seconds)
    rotational exercises on page 159.

Strengthening
    Curl-ups
    Side push-ups
    Prone off table, coming up into extension
    Side bridge
    Back bridge with pillows under sknee
    Push-ups in parallel bars (standing)

Pole exercises (3) done with pole across shoulders behind neck, one hand at each end:
1. Right hand will go to left foot, return upright.
   Left hand will go to right foot, return upright.
2. Right hand will go toward right knee as patient bends sideways.
   Repeat on the left.
3. Patient will turn pole toward the rear, turning at the waist only.
   Return to front and repeat on the other side.

PRE's
    Chop and lift patterns with wall pulleys
    Duplicate any other movements that can be isolated from patient's sport

Gait
    Patient will use mirror to correct gait
    Patient will learn to move to music to regain normal movement of body

Cardiovascular Fitness
Progressively run stairs, to patient's tolerance, increasing daily.
Stationary bicycle
1 mile light tension
1 mile heavy tension

Correct body mechanics
to be practiced during sport movements

Limbering

Relaxation

The patient remained on his functional program for one month before beginning to swim, and then he used the relaxation, limbering, and flexibility as warm-up and cool-down exercises.

After two and a half months of therapy the only remaining limitation the patient experienced was the inability to sit for long periods of time without developing stiffness. He was advised to change positions before that happened. The height of his desk and chair was checked. His daily posture was examined. And finally, he was given a relaxation program to perform at his desk periodically during the day. The patient has reported back several times during the past year and has had no exacerbations of low-back pain or limitations.

POSTLAMINECTOMY TREATMENT

Patient #4 was four days postlaminectomy, and complained of pain in her back while lying in her hospital bed. She was 45 years old, and an active woman who had experienced low-back pain for 5 years prior to surgery.

After evaluating the patient, it was evident that she was experiencing spasm on both sides of her back. The paraspinal muscles were hard and tight, and tender to palpation. Movement was difficult and painful.

With the suture line covered, the patient received ethyl chloride spray to the muscles in spasm. Under these conditions the amount of spray must be at the therapist's discretion and not by the patient's report of burning, pain, etc., because of the decreased sensation present due to the incision.

When the pain had subsided enough so that she could roll onto her back, the patient was taught breathing, relaxation, and limbering exercises. This treatment was repeated several times daily until the sutures were removed. At that time the patient came to the physical therapy department and received electric stimulation, ice pack (20 minutes), followed by the same exercise routine with the addition of pelvic tilt 1 and LBS1 with the assistance of the therapist.

Once the spasm was broken and the patient had regained enough of her general strength and normal movement, she was given a Kraus-Weber muscle test and a flexibility test. Ambulation was begun in the therapeutic pool, and her program was constructed in the manner stated above.

The movements to be avoided during the first eight weeks of treatment are repetitive bending and rotation under stress. Of course, no heavy lifting is permitted. After two months, however, if the patient has made substantial progress, there should be no restrictions put upon the patient. Pain should be the best guide to what should be avoided. However, it is not uncommon for a postlaminectomy patient to feel an aching and pulling, as scar tissue is being stretched for several months after surgery, and this should not be misconstrued as pain. Any numbness or weakness that was present before surgery will also take several weeks or months to disappear.

After three months of physical therapy treatments the patient was able to switch to a functional program and to daily swimming. Now, six months postsurgery, she has resumed her active life of wife, mother, and career-woman.

VERTEBRAL INSTABILITY

Patient #5 was an ex-athlete, and had suffered intermittent back pain for a period of 6 years. The pain had begun after his athletic career had ended. He was 35 years old and in good "all around" condition. His muscular strength was normal, except for the abdominals. However, his flexibility was not, as was indicated by his fingertips being 15 inches from the floor in HS4 exercise. The pain sometimes radiated into one buttock or the other, and on occasion there was sciatic pain.

Vertebral instability can be caused by disc degeneration or trauma or both, and usually produces a strain or irritation of the posterior facet joint. This can cause pain local to the back or pain that radiates, which can be easily confused with sciatica, as this patient experienced periodically.

There was no spasm upon evaluating this patient; however, he was supplied with the necessary information should one occur in the future. He was started on a program to induce relaxation and increases flexibility. After two weeks the patient was taught two exercises that add natural traction through active mobilization to the vertebral column, which, in turn, relieves stress on the posterior joints and discs. The two exercises are LBS4 and P1. P1 is done with a slight variation for this purpose. The patient assumes the position described in P1 and, while holding the pelvic tilt, also pushes the back of the neck into the mat. The patient continues to push both his back and neck into the mat while counting to six, and while continuing to breathe naturally.

As an added precaution, abdominal and low-back strengthening exercises were also added. Additionally, the patient was advised to avoid forward stooping, arching of the back, or maintaining any work position with hands overhead, as all of these positions will encourage hyperextension sprains.

A year and a half later, Patient #5 is able to continue enjoying sporting activities by performing his exercise program daily, and before and after strenuous activity. He was cautioned on positions to eliminate and how to apply proper body mechanics during movement.

POSTSURGERY (15 YEARS)

Patient #6 is a 60-year-old active and outgoing woman who experienced her initial attack of back pain in 1960 and was admitted to a nearby hospital. She remained an in-patient for 3 months and received the standard conservative treatment for a HNP, such as bedrest, traction, anti-inflammatory drugs, and analgesics. This treatment was not successful and the patient underwent L_5-S_1 discectomy and laminectomy. She received no follow-up physical therapy after surgery.

In the time span of 15 years following surgery to the time of her first patient assessment (2 years ago), this patient experienced 25 hospital admissions because of pain on the right side of her back. Each time she was treated with bedrest, traction, and medication.

Two years ago she was evaluated just after a painful episode of back pain had ended. She was 15 inches from the floor in doing exercise HS4, and had weak abdominals and low-back muscles. On the right she had weak (F) hip abductor and big toe extensor. Right ankle dorsiflexion was good. She experienced numbness at the back of the right calf, lateral heel, foot, and toe. Functionally, she could not roll up to a sitting position, and also had difficulty reclining, and coming up from the floor. Bending to pick up an object from the floor was nearly impossible, and she was fearful of lifting or carrying objects.

The patient was instructed in relaxation and limbering exercises, to be preceded by a hot bath, as long as no spasm was present. As soon as the pain had decreased, exercises such as LBS6, LBS1, and P1 were added. When the patient had gained some of her mobility without pain, other flexibility exercises were added. Gradually, the strengthening exercises were added. Several months later the patient was once again checked, and was found to have increased flexibility (fingertips to the floor) and good muscle strength in all muscle groups.

The patient was not seen again for 2 years, but by her explanation of events, she had no exacerbations until about a year and a half later after which time she had stopped her exercises for a period of a few months. Again, the patient was reevaluated, and it found that flexibility had decreased in the low-back area, and the abdominals had decreased back to "2." This was the best motivation possible, as the patient, herself, observed that while on an exercise program she could carry out her daily activities, but once she stopped exercising, the pain and mobility limitations returned. She requested another exercise program, and is currently using it daily to prevent future episodes. Information on icing and general relaxation techniques was also provided.

The patient was also taught to do two additional exercises that would increase mobility of the vertebra through *active mobilization* and stretch the trunk muscle in a rotary pattern rather than a straight plane. Since she had been pain free for several months, rotational exercises were entirely permissable for this patient, and they did not cause "aches" or "pains" while she performed them. The exercises are pictured on the following page.

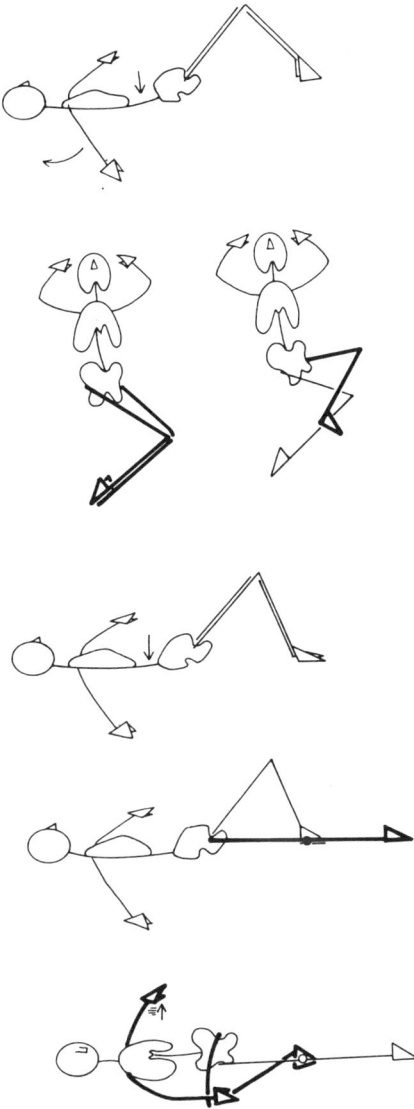

As soon as her full flexibility returns, she will carefully practice rolling, sitting, reclining to the floor and returning upright, and carrying and lifting objects in order to prevent further strain.

This patient is a good example of how physical therapy treatment can be used adequately as Preventive Medicine. Had she received the exercise program and education on how to manage muscle spasm during the postsurgery period, most likely she would not have needed an additional 25 hospital admissions, and the waste in time, effort, and money would not have occurred.

LIGAMENT SPRAIN

Patient #7 was a 21-year-old young man who was injured 2 days earlier during a football game. Since that time he had experienced extreme pain in the low-back area, and his general mobility and movement was limited. The physician diagnosed muscle spasm with probable ligament sprain.

He received ice packs for 30 minutes across the low back, followed by 10 minutes of low tetanizing current, and 10 minutes of surging current. Breathing, relaxation, and gentle limbering exercises were taught. The patient was fitted with a back support to be worn continuously, except for treatment time, during the acute state only (7 to 10 days) for the purpose of restricting his movements.

Once the spasm had ended, the patient was evaluated once again. There was pain on palpation over the supraspinous ligament and over the tip of the spinous process where the ligament attaches, at vertebra L_4-L_5. Active flexion of the back in the forward flexed position and passive hyperflexion of the spine duplicated the patient's pain, whereas passive extension and active hyperextension were pain-free.

The patient continued with the same treatment (except for the change to 15 minutes surging current and heat, once the spasm was broken) for 2 weeks. At that time the patient was pain-free, except for a slight ache in the hyperflexed position, and was found to have normal muscle strength except for the low-back muscles, and a lack of flexibility in hamstrings, calf, low back, and hip flexor muscles. He was put on a functional exercise program of breathing, relaxation, limbering, flexibility, strengthening, and body mechanics to be practiced during running, football, etc. During the exercise program he was cautioned to continue to avoid the extreme forward flexion position for another 2 weeks. In 4 weeks he returned to football with no exacerbations.

TREATMENT COMPONENTS

The idea of treatment components is introduced so that therapists would be exposed to two concepts: first, so that a method would be presented that would allow therapists to logically match a treatment component to the patient's symptoms, and secondly, so that different levels of treatment could be recognized and a corresponding treatment program could be appropriately constructed by the therapists. These two concepts are important in applying the Low-Back Exercise Program detailed in this book, because within the structure of the program there is great flexibility that the therapists can use at their discretion to the patient's advantage.

For example, if a patient presents with a muscle spasm that is aggravated by the specific treatment outlined in Chap. 4, therapists have many options open to them if they consider the Component concept. They can ice before or after the electric stimulation. Or, they may change the manner in which they applied electric stimulation. If the patient finds tetanizing curent too painful even after icing, they may try a low surging current only. The treatment modalities that are presented in Chap. 4 are ideally what is best to treat the diagnosed symptom/condition, but they should be modified to meet the needs of the individual patient.

If a patient refuses an injection for a triggerpoint, the physician may recommend either friction-type massage with the thumb or ultrasound (pulsed) for their mechanical effect on the triggerpoint. Icing can precede the friction massage to reduce the accompanying pain, whereas heat would be a better adjunct to ultrasound therapy. In some cases the patient may find a large ice pack too uncomfortable, but will be able to tolerate ice massage over the involved muscle, and specifically over the triggerpoint. With an older patient, you may find that they refuse any attempts at icing. However, therapists must make every effort to convince the patients of the importance of ice therapy during the treatment of the spasm only. If they cannot tolerate the ice directly, several hot towels may be spread over the patient's back before application of the ice. This lessens the initial shock of the cold. Or, a thin layer of a moisturizing cream may be gently applied to the area before being sprayed with ethyl chloride. Once the spasm is broken, however, ice need no longer be used for pain if the patient's tolerance to it is low. Any one of the different forms of heat may precede the treatment and occasionally will be of some benefit in reducing pain. The transcutaneous nerve stimulator is a very useful modality to reduce pain and to allow the patient to progress through his exercise program. However, the physician must have first ascertained that the chronic pain the patient is experiencing is not from any other serious pathology, but is chronic low-back pain only. The placement of the electrodes usually requires some experimentation for each patient, but once this is established, the TNS is another noninvasive technique that is very successful for the control of pain.

Therapists can make the Component concept work for them if they first list the main problems from the Patient Assessment, and then choose the correct components to treat the symptom/condition. If the initial choice of components does not assist the patient sufficiently, therapists should take advantage of the flexibility within the low-back Exercise Program, and formulate another treatment program in conjunction with the physician.

Table 2 shows contraindications to be observed during treatment.

Table 2. Contraindications During Treatment

Symptom or Condition	Contraindication
Muscle spasm	Stretching
Increased muscle tension	Exercise without general relaxation
Lack of flexibility	Overstretching
Muscle weakness	Strain
Triggerpoints	Vigorous contractions or overstretching of affected muscle
Ligamentous sprain	Unnecessary stress first 2 weeks
Muscle strain	High-repetition exercises Vigorous exercise too early
Facet dysfunction	Rotation with flexion Hyperextension sprains
Nerve Root { Tension, Irritation, Compression }	During Acute Stage { Stretching of sciatica, Rotation with flexion } Hyperextension Sprains
Spondylolisthesis	Hyperextension sprains Complete forward flexion Jerky or quick twisting movements
Scoliosis	Same as facet dysfunction
Increased lumbar lordosis	Hyperextension Overstretching of hamstrings Elimination of hamstring strengthening
Compression fracture	Unnecessary stress first 2 weeks
Osteoporosis	Inactivity

Table 2. (continued)

Symptom or Condition	Contraindication
Osteoarthritis	Exercises with high repetitions Unnecessary strain on joints
Laminectomies	SLR and pelvic tilts for 2 weeks Repetitive forward flexion Rotation with stress Heavy lifting After 8 weeks, all else permitted
Fusion	Foward flexion until fusion is solid

SUMMARY

Lengthy investigation and research by Kraus and Weber indicate that 80% of back pain is produced by accumulated muscular tension due to increased stress and strain of living in an exercise-deficient society. The purpose of beginning each exercise program with breathing, relaxation, and limbering exercises is to teach patients "how" to relax by ridding themselves of this tension, and to prepare them mentally and physically for the ensuing exercise regime. Each program is ended with the same gentle exercises, also, so that the working muscles will be returned to their resting physiological state after having been contracted during specific exercises.

During the early stages of the treatment the elimination of pain is the goal and this is, of course, enough motivation in itself for the emotionally healthy patient. During the maintainence-oriented programs, motivation should be geared toward individual ADL activities. Patients should always know and understand why they are performing specific movements and exercises and how these exercises relate to their functional capacity. The motivation during functionally oriented programs is to be able to perform the skill of their sport without pain and limitation. Isolated movements from the patients sport should be included within the treatment program. In order for therapists to be successful in motivating any patient, they first must know at what level the patients are presently capable of performing, and present them with a short-term goal that is reachable. Therapists must give patients the necessary guidance and confidence to reach the goal with exercises that are separate entities of the total movement. Patients must be kept in an active role at all times; they must know their goal, and the steps available to reach it.

Chapter 6

Body Movement and Mechanics

When instructing the patient in proper body movement and mechanics, the therapist will do well to remember that one must consider both the forces working on the skeletal system (and disc) and the separate demands put on the muscular system. Sometimes these forces oppose one another, and during the early stages of rehabilitation both the therapist and the patient must often make a choice as to what position to assume. This differentiation of posture is extremely important if there is a deficit in either system, such as muscle deficiencies or discogenic pathology. An example of this is shown in Fig. 7. Using the curl-up position, it is evident that placement of the arms easily changes the distance between the axis of motion and the center of gravity. The gravitational force increases proportionately as this distance increases. Therefore, a maximum contraction of the abdominals would be required to maintain the patient's body in position 7b, and is definitely an exercise that would be effective in strengthening the abdominals. This same curl-up, however, is often used by the therapist in assisting a patient with acute pain to the sitting position or in rolling over. However, Nachemson reports (Fig. 8) that the curl-up position represents the exercise position that puts the most strain on the patients back by raising the intradiscal pressure (at L_3) to the highest level in relation to all other current exercises used in rehabilitating the low back patient.

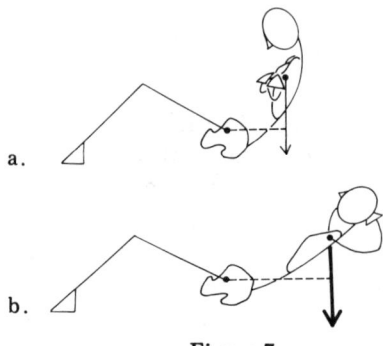

Figure 7.

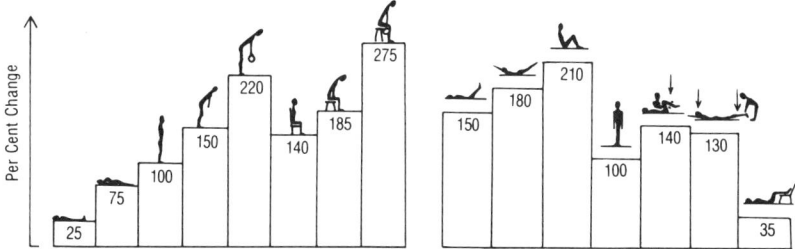

Figure 8. Relative changes in pressure (or load) in the third lumbar disc of living subjects (a) in various positions and (b) in various muscle-strengthening exercises. From SPINE 1:59-71, M1976. Copyright © 1976. Medical Department, Harper & Row, Publishers, Inc., Hagerstown, MD.

This is not to say that the curl-up exercise should not be used with low-back patients, but it does mean that the therapist must know how and when to use it as a therapeutic exercise. The position should be eliminated entirely in patients who exhibit acute symptoms of a HNP, compression on a nerve, or nerve root irritation.

If the patient does not exhibit serious symptoms in either system, then one general scheme of proper body positioning, movement, and mechanics emerges as the proper one according to scientific and technological information available. Methods of preventing injury to the back in the healthy subject (4a) is the same as the methods presented to the patient who has suffered back pain and injury in the past, but is now rehabilitated to the level of the healthy subject (4). Otherwise, proper movement is taught in steps to patients who have lost the "feeling" for natural movements [(2) and (3)], because they have not moved naturally for long periods of time due to either pain or limitation of movement for other reasons.

Here is a continuum that explains this concept:

Subject	(4a) Healthy Subject	(1) Spasm or triggerpoint	(2) Muscular deficiency	(3) Skeletal etiology disc vs instability Hyperextension sprain	(4) Healthy subject (Rehabilitated)
Goal of proper body mechanics	Prevention of back injury	Avoidance of aggravating situations	Prevention of muscle strain	Mechanical unloading of the back	Prevention of future episodes

SPASM OR TRIGGERPOINT (1)

The patient who is experiencing a muscle spasm or who is receiving postinjection treatment is taught how to avoid aggravating positions. Rather than being taught proper body mechanics, this patient is taught proper posture and body movements. The patient must learn to support his or her back protectively so as to avoid future strain to an area that is not yet prepared to accept it. Positions and conditions that keep or return the muscles to a shortened state, such as general tension, high repetition movements, and constant postures, should be avoided. Here is a more detailed guide:

Symptom/Condition	Guide to Proper Posture and Body Movement
Spasm Post-triggerpoint injection treatment	Change positions frequently Do not sit, stand, or walk for more than 30 minutes at a time When sitting, rest the feet on a stool to raise flexed knees higher than hips When standing, raise the foot on the painful side on a stool or whatever else is available Avoid exertion Avoid stressful situations Avoid any repetitous movements from day-to-day routine (such as reaching in one direction, twisting to one side) Avoid any activities that cause pain Do not travel long distances Avoid any form of transportation that can cause quick, jerky movements. Sleep on a hard mattress and/or bedboard Sexual intercourse should be avoided during acute spasm only. Two proper bed positions: 1. Supine with one pillow under the neck and two pillows supporting back of knees 2. On either side with knees bent up. The top knee should surpass the bottom one, and rest on a pillow that is on top of the bottom knee Proper treatment position: Prone, with one or two pillows under the abdomen, depending on the patient's anatomy. Enough support should be given so that the strain is relieved and the lordosis is relaxed. A pillow should also support the dorsal aspect of the feet. The patient may or may not request a pillow under the head.

The therapist should reassure the patient that most of these limitations are for a short time only, and as soon as the spasm has ended, or the triggerpoint dissolved, he or she will be able to return to more normal activities by relearning natural movements that were lost because of pain. Constant reminders of this will make it easier for the patient to accept these limitations.

This period of treatment is usually the only time that a patient's lifestyle is so limited because of pain or disability, unless severe limitations exist in muscle strength, flexibility, or mobility. Most patients, however, will have had some muscular abnormalities and pain for a period of time prior to the acute episode and will have lost some basic "feeling" for natural movements. These patients should not be discharged from the rehabilitation program until all functional movements on the assessment sheet can be performed fluidly and in a coordinated manner, as demonstrated in the following section.

MUSCULAR DEFICIENCY (2)

The patient who presents with muscular deficiency (2), but without either spasm or triggerpoint symptoms, is in a very vulnerable state. The original, acute pain is no longer present, and does not act as a reminder of the patient's limitations during normal daily activities. Therefore, the therapist must teach proper body mechanics to this patient with special emphasis on protective body control and positioning, because even normal movements could cause strain to a patient with muscle deficiency.

An example of this would be if the patient is taught to roll from supine to sidelying: A protective movement would be for the patient to roll his or her entire body at once, instead of first dropping the knees to one side and then continuing to roll. A patient with normal muscle strength could easily roll from supine to sidelying by first dropping the knees to one side, without injuring any skeletal, or supporting muscular, components. However, without this normal muscular support, muscular or skeletal strain is possible.

The following movements are presented with this type of protection for the patient with muscular deficiency in mind. The patient must perform these movements many times while consciously being aware of the crucial points of using the entire body and gravity to his advantage, rather than just the back to assist with the movement. This continuous repetition of proper body movement with conscious control will soon produce effective carryover into the patient's lifestyle, and then they will become effortless, coordinated movements that look "natural." Even the patient will often remark that "It feels good to be able to move again."

The following five principles are constant throughout all movements and should be kept in mind at all times by both the patient and the therapist:

1. The chin should be tucked on the chest, and hands and arms kept as close to the body as possible. In this manner the stress on the back is kept at a minimum by decreasing the distance the center of gravity must move away from the fixed fulcrum represented by the L/S joint.

2. The abdominal muscles should be contracted at the time of movement. This adds a natural splint to the back by causing the back extensors to contract at the same time to add an equal but opposing force to the one created by the original contraction of the abdominals. The patient may also be taught to forcefully exhale from the abdomen while beginning the movement if there is difficulty with an appropriate contraction of the abdominals. The forcible exhalation will automatically contract the abdominals, and thus, the back extensors.

3. When moving to the upright position, the patient should use a downward force whenever possible in order to take advantage of Newton's third law, which describes a force equal in magnitude but opposite in direction, to assist in the desired movement. An example would be when the patient wishes to come to the standing position from the sitting position from a chair, he or she should push downward, firmly, on his knees to use his body strength, and gravity, to their utmost in assisting his movement.

4. The body should always be moved as a unit. Whenever flexion is required, it should come from the hips, and not the vertebral column. An example of this would be when the patient wishes to stand from a chair, he leans forward from the hips to place his hands on his knees, rather than "hunching" his back forward.

5. Whenever the patient wishes to twist or turn, the movement should originate and occur at the level of the feet and legs and hips. No rotation should take place at the thoracic or lumbar region.

BODY MOVEMENTS

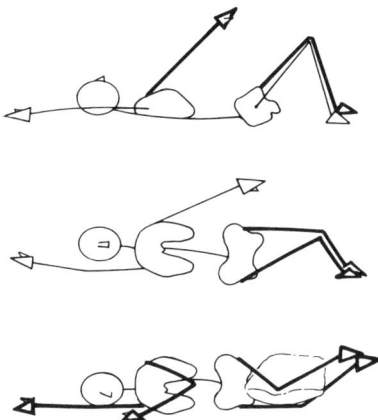

Supine to side-lying—supine with knees bent, feet flat. Right hand should be outstretched overhead. The patient will be rolling to the right side. Raise left hand and arm straight up to the ceiling, parallel with the knees. Let knees and left arm roll together to right side. This will allow the body to move as a unit. Knees will be on the floor and bent up toward the chest. The head will be on top of the right arm that is still overhead. If the patient wishes to stay in this position, two pillows should be provided for under the head, and one for between the knees. The uppermost knee should slightly surpass the bottom knee and rest on the pillow.

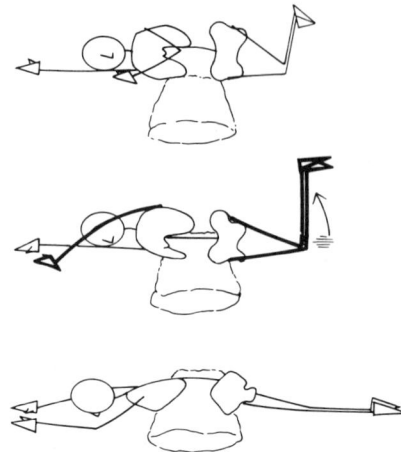

Side-lying to prone—continue to roll from side-lying position so that both the left knee and forearm are also touching the floor. The knees should be squeezed together during the roll to prevent the legs from "flopping" and twisting the back. They should be bent throughout the roll. The patient should roll onto a pillow to be placed under the abdomen.

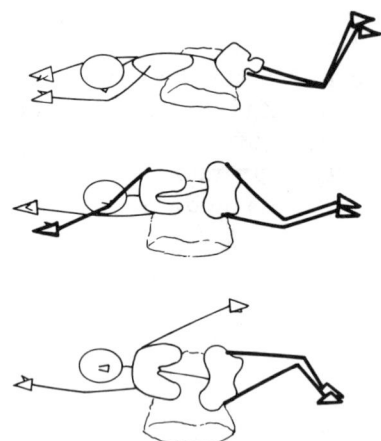

Prone back to supine—bend both knees and squeeze them together. Lift the left arm overhead, and while pushing the right ear into the pillow (or the right arm if there is no pillow), roll both knees and left arm over at once. This will keep the body as a unit as the patient rolls onto the back.

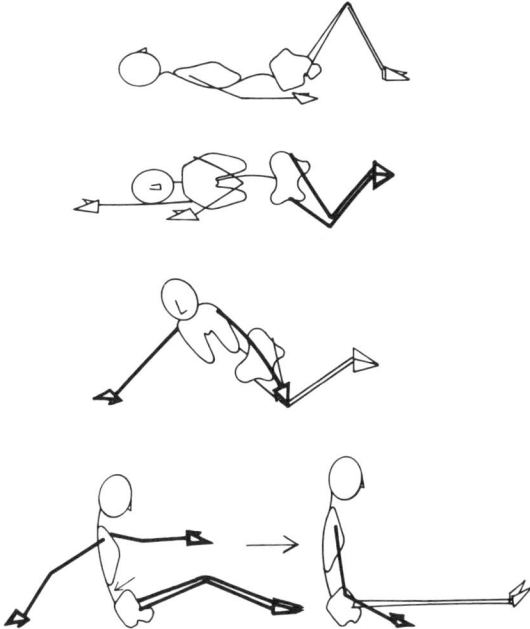

Supine to Side-Sitting—supine with knees bent, feet flat. Roll to the side-lying as described above, ending with knees on the floor, bent up to the chest. The right arm is extended overhead, and the left palm is on the floor in front of the right shoulder. While pushing down hard with the left hand the body weight will shift over the left hand while the right hand is also placed palm down as close to the body as possible. Both hands are pushing down, while the chin is tucked and the stomach is pulled in, the patient moves to an upright sitting position. This is the side-sitting position and can be a prelude to the long-sitting position by just having the patient move the right hand in closer to the body while the left hand and arm turn with the knees so that both buttocks are on the floor. The patient may retain the sitting position with the knees bent, or the long-sitting position by extending the legs. Or, the side-sitting position may be used to help the patient get up from the plinthe or bed as described on the following page.

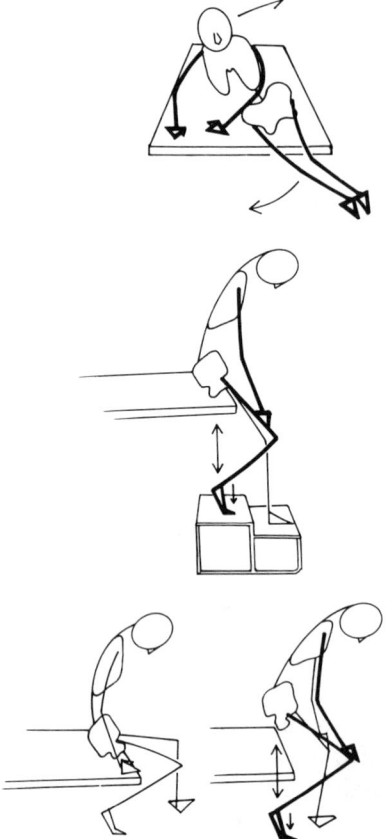

Supine to side-sitting to getting up from plinthe or bed—the patient should be as close as possible to the edge of the bed or plinthe for this exercise. The patient assumes the side-sitting position as described above, and pivots on the right buttock so that as both legs drop off the edge, the top part of the body assumes the upright position, ending on both buttocks, and in the sitting position without straining the back. If the plinthe is high, a step stool can be placed nearby so the patient can place the right foot on the top step and the left on the step below (if the stool is high enough) and raise up by straightening the knees and lifting the buttocks off the plinthe, and not be bending from the back. When assuming the upright position from sitting, it is always better to have the right foot underneath, or as close to the buttocks as possible, as this adds better leverage to the motion by moving the pivot point closer to the body. The patient should be instructed to push the right foot down into the stool, which will in turn raise the buttocks up from the plinthe. If the bed is of average height, the patient can slide to the edge so that the right foot with toes bent into the floor can be placed slightly under the bed and under the buttocks, and continue as above.

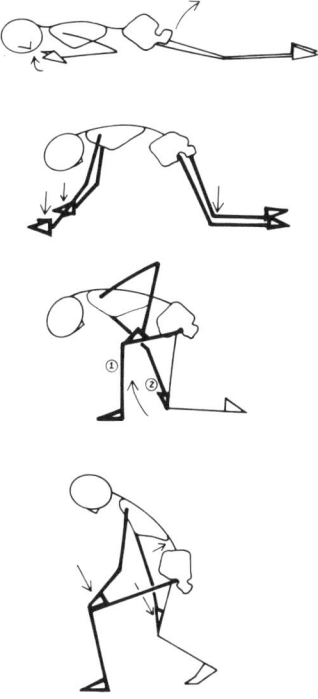

Prone to hands and knees to standing—remove pillows and bring the hands underneath shoulders being careful not to arch the back. Keep chin tucked, stomach pulled in. While pushing hands and knees into the bed, the body will raise up. The knees will act as a pivot point. Take the left knee up toward the chest and place the foot on the floor to stand. The left hand pushes downward on the left knee while the chin is tucked and stomach is pulled in. The right hand is placed on the right knee, which is still on the floor. Most of the body weight is over right heel, and it will shift to the middle (between both feet) when the patient pushes downward with both hands. The slight twist that takes place is not from the back but is produced from the transferring of the weight from right side to middle. As the weight shifts the patient will place the right foot on the floor, and by pushing downward with both hands on both knees, will assume the upright position by extending both knees.

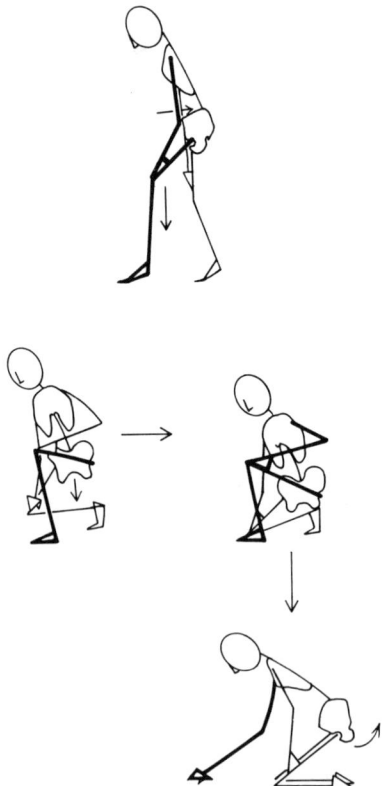

Standing to hands and knees—take a step forward with the left foot and allow the left hand to slide down to the left knee by flexing slightly at the hips. Pull in stomach and press down on left knee and right thigh with right hand. Right knee goes to floor, and toes are bent, and ball of foot rests on floor. Reach for floor with right hand, not by bending back but by lifting buttocks off the right foot. Put left hand and knee on the floor.

Body Movement and Mechanics 175

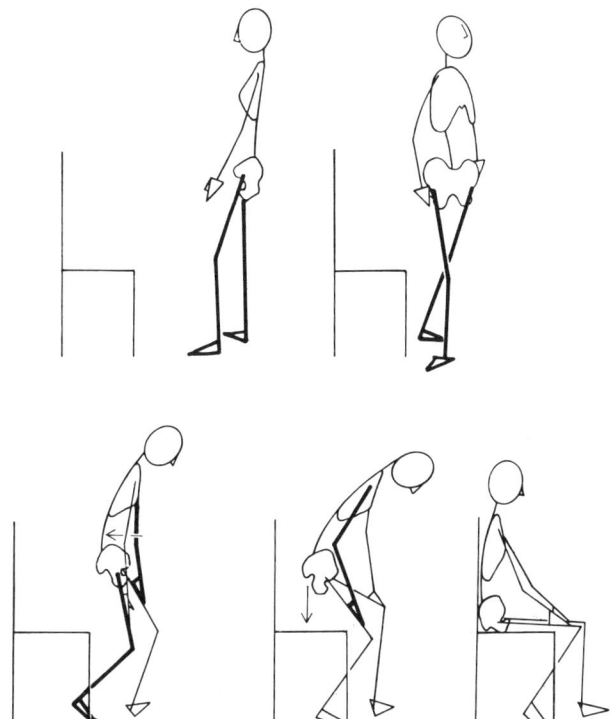

Standing to sitting in chair—walk to chair. Turn to bring your back to chair by pivoting on feet and not by twisting back. Step back with right foot, left foot is in front. Slide left hand to left knee by lowering the buttocks and by slightly flexing at the hips. While keeping chin tucked and stomach pulled in, lower self to chair resting hands on knees and lowering buttocks by bending knees.

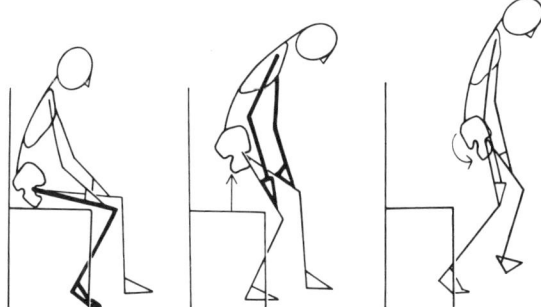

Sitting to standing—left foot will be in front of right. Right foot is under chair as much as possible. Lean forward by lifting buttocks by pushing down hard with both hands. Keep chin tucked and abdominals tightened. Pinch buttocks to assume pelvic tilt while coming to the standing position.

These activities are just an example of the many ADL movements that can be constructed by the therapist by keeping in mind the five principles for safe movement given at the beginning of this chapter. The occupational therapist is in an opportune position to both teach and reinforce proper body posture and movement in the hospital-setting. Oftentimes, their contact with the patient is in a more relaxed and less stressful environment, and these conditions are generally more conducive to a true learning experience. Group sessions under these conditions with an occupational therapist pointing out the proper way to sit down into a chair, the proper posture to assume during treatment time, and, again, how to stand from the chair when the treatment has ended, would be excellent reinforcement of proper body posture and movement.

Most times the role of the occupational therapist is overlooked when considering the total rehabilitation approach to the low-back patient. Their true importance, however, is revealed when the patient is finally ready to apply the new postures, both mental and physical, to a healthy activity which will be a true test of the patients functional capabilities. Constant repetition of the patient's proper body posture and movements will develop proprioceptive and kinesthetic senses so that soon the patient will perform the movements "naturally" and without having to think about each step of the movement. Eventually, patients will develop the skill in movement and the confidence in their abilities necessary to return safely to the lifestyle of their choice.

SKELETAL ETIOLOGY (3)

Patients who experience pain from a skeletal etiology must accept a more defensive attitude toward their disability. They must admit that their problem will be long-standing, even though the acute symptoms may subside, and that certain compromises must be made in their life. The main goal of these patients' preventive program will be to teach them how to mechanically unload the back of all unnecessary forces and to prevent strains by regulating the types of activities they will participate in. Heavy lifting, contact sports, and other activities that call for the patient to remain in the "bent-over" position repetitively, or for any length of time, must be eliminated. Flexion of the back with rotation against resistance must also be guarded against.

Although increased muscle strength will protect the patient to some degree, the original skeletal etiology will still exist, and will continue to be a potential hazard if the patient disregards his condition. Therefore, patient education is of the utmost importance here, and is one of the main responsibilities of the therapist. Here are some guidelines to consider:

Symptom/Condition	Guide to mechanically unloading the back
	The patient
"Disc"	Must learn to decrease the forces acting on the back by decreasing the lumbar lordosis (Fig. 9)
Vertebral instability	
Hyperextension sprain	
	May require the temporary use of a corset to:
	help achieve a normal curve
	decrease the lordosis
	add additional abdominal support
	decrease posterior intradiscal pressure
	decrease mobility
	reduce the need for spasm (which is the natural splinting action of the back)
	Must perform abdominal strengthening exercises;
	isometric exercises and pelvic tilting, both with and without neck push, are appropriate
	May have to lose weight if necessary
	Should avoid general fatigue

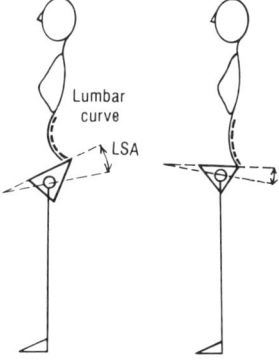

Figure 9. (a) Increased lordosis caused by bad posture. (b) Decreased lordosis achieved by proper positioning and mechanically unloading the back.

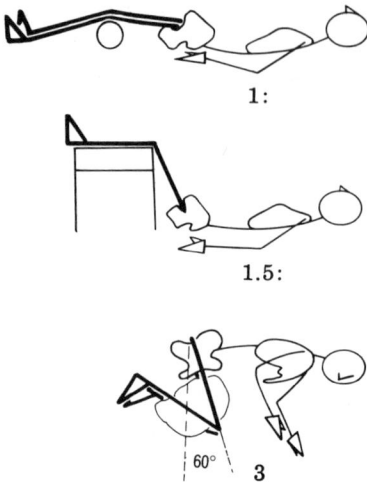

Figure 10. Acceptable positions of rest and their corresponding ratio of intradiscal pressure: (a) supine with knees slightly bent on pillow or towel; (b) supine with knees bent to 90° supported by a stool; (c) sidelying with hips and knees bent.

The contradiction of forces on the skeletal system and muscular considerations is again evident in the pictured positions of rest (Fig. 10). As the ratio of intradiscal pressure rises by the changes in position, there is a corresponding increase in the stretch put on the paravertebral muscles. For a patient who is experiencing muscle tightness or is trying to avoid reoccurring spasms, position 10c would be most beneficial. Although there is a proportion increase in intradiscal pressure, the patient who does present with these symptoms should be advised to assume the sidelying, with hips and knees bent, position (with pillow between knees), because the benefits are considered to outweigh disadvantages. Actually, any of the pictured rest positions are acceptable for the patient experiencing back pain.

In the early stages of rehabilitation the patient should avoid exercises which would

1. stretch the sciatica, such as hamstring stretches and positions where the head and knees are raised concurrently (Fig. 11);
2. cause hyperextension sprains (Fig. 12) by returning to the extended position against resistance, by sustaining a

force while in rotation and slight flexion, or by performing strenuous exercises or movements with the back in hyperextension;

3. raise intradiscal pressure, such as the curl-up, and its variations (Fig. 13).

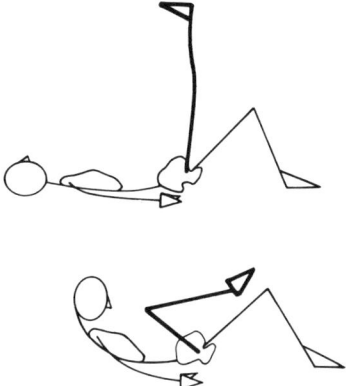

Figure 11.

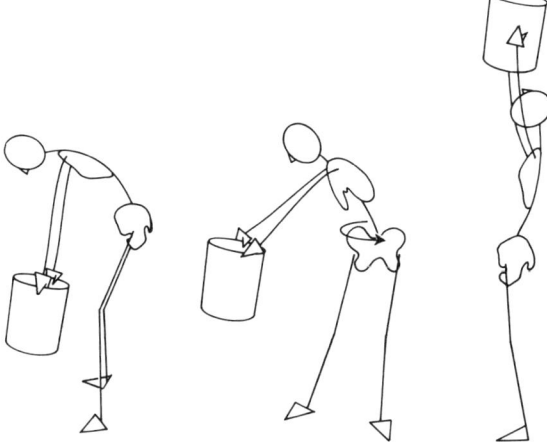

Figure 12.

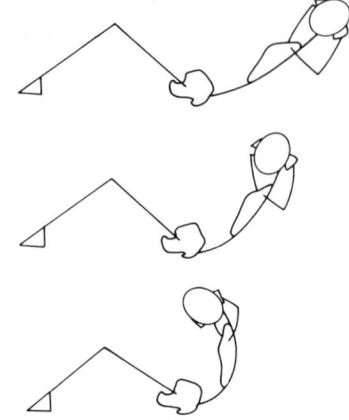

Figure 13.

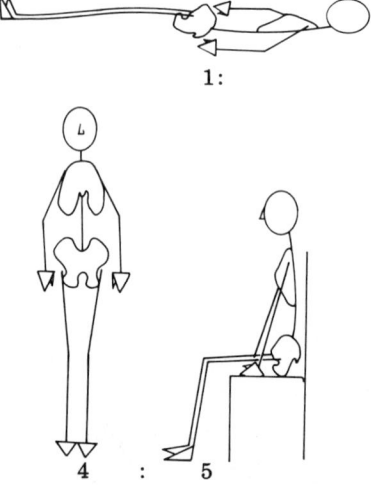

Figure 14. Ratio representing the relationship of the intradiscal pressure resulting from position changes.

Figure 14 shows the need for bedrest with a patient with an acute HNP, and, also, why many patients with "discs" find it difficult, or even impossible, to sit. The waiting rooms of many back clinics are filled with patients who stand, or pace the floor, while waiting for their appointments. The intradiscal pressure in sitting is five times that of pressure in the reclining position.

As the patient's body moves away from the y axis, and the angle of movement increases, there is more stress put on the lumbar discs and

Body Movement and Mechanics

the lumbosacral junction. In Fig. 15c, the patient is erect and there is no angle deviating from the y axis, therefore, the only force acting on the patient's back is a downward compression force, which is equal to the patient's weight. In contrast, Fig. 15a and 15b demonstrate the increases in force applied to the back in the "bent-over" position.

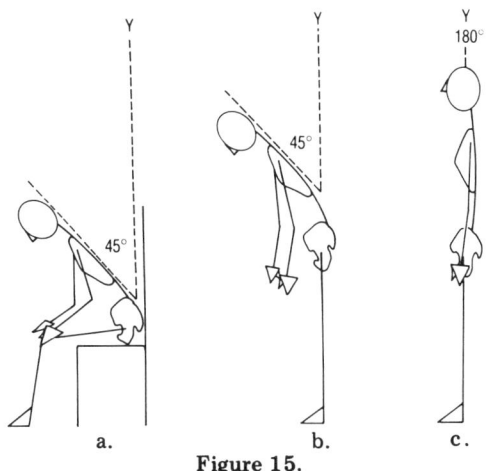

Figure 15.

It is evident, then, that body posture, positioning, and movement is of utmost importance to the patient suffering from a symptomatic "disc." In the initial period of therapy, skeletal considerations always outweigh muscular ones, and for the most part, the therapist will have to consider carefully positioning and force changes affecting the back, when requesting the patient to participate in physical therapy. The back must be "mechanically unloaded" whenever possible.

When the patient has remained symptom-free for two to three months he can be considered a (Rehabilitated) Healthy Subject, and relearn how to perform the movements presented in the following section.

PREVENTION OF BACK INJURY FOR THE HEALTHY SUBJECT (4, 4a)

Muscular Considerations

Keeping the muscles of the body both flexible and strong are the first prerequisites for avoiding an episode of back pain. Although all muscles require these two components for efficient operation, flexibility will be most important in the paravertebral, hamstrings, and the hip flexors. Strength will be most important in the abdominals and upper and lower back muscles (including gluteals).

Patients who have already experienced their first episode of back pain must remain on their maintanence program indefinitely, especially if they live a sedentary life. Others who have not yet experienced serious back pain must also be tested and put on a preventive exercise program. Even patients who engage in strenuous sports should be tested from time to time, as weaknesses in the back and abdominals are often found even in athletes. No one is exempt from the hazard of back injury and back pain, but patients who practice relaxation to relieve excess tension and shortening of the muscles, plus flexiblity and strengthening exercises, will be providing themselves maximum protection.

If a patient wishes to practice a sport, he or she should be on a conditioning (or functional) program for one to two months before working out in the sport. This program should include relaxation, limbering, flexibility, and strengthening components, especially of the muscles to be subjected to the most use during the activity. As many movements as possible should be extrapolated from the sport and duplicated using proper body movements and mechanics, in the presence of the therapist. If possible, the therapist should be with the patient the first two or three times he practices the sport, to correct any faulty postures. The longer a patient practices a faulty movement, the more it becomes a habit, and the more difficult it is to break.

An example would be in transferring a patient from a conditioning (or functional) program to a swimming exercise. Unless the patient has had prior training in swimming and is an excellent swimmer, he or she will probably kick from the knees and keep his head in the extended position while doing the crawl. To strengthen the back and gluteal muscles he or she should be instructed to keep the knees extended while kicking. Also, if the patient does not have the proper head position, he or she is likely to assume an increased lordosis and a constant (straining) contraction of the back extensors. The head should be in slight flexion to prevent this. If the therapist does not have a deep enough understanding of the sport, the patient should be advised to obtain instruction from a professional instructor.

Of the three most popular swim strokes, the crawl, the breast stroke, and the side stroke, the crawl is the best stroke for the patient first embarking on a swimming program. The side stroke requires the use of the same muscles constantly, and without a chance for relaxation of the working muscle between strokes, whereas with the crawl the muscles are worked alternately and neither side is held in a constant contraction. The hazard with the breast stroke is that beginners and even intermediate swimmers tend to arch the back as they lift the head to breathe. When the patient has been swimming the crawl for two months, symptom-free, he or she can consider the other strokes after receiving qualified instruction in technique.

The patient should use the relaxation, limbering, and flexibility exercises as a warm-up before and a cool-down after swimming. The entire conditioning (or functional) program should be performed on the days the patient does not swim.

Relaxation

Relaxation training is important for all patients. For those whose etiology of pain is of a muscular origin, removing excess tension from skeletal muscles will also remove much of the pain. It will relieve tight muscles, and, consequently, will relieve the susceptibility of muscle spasm, lack of flexibility, and a multitude of other possible problems. For patients suffering from pain from a skeletal etiology, relaxation training will remove the aggravating muscle tightness and/or imbalance that can precipitate an acute episode. Pain that a patient "must live with" can also be controlled or abated through relaxation techniques.

The first thing a patient must learn is how to get in touch with his body by learning how to coordinate mind and body "togetherness." For some it will be an entirely new experience, while for others it will be a return to a more relaxed, healthy, and happy state of mind and body that the patient had experienced at other times in his life. The two most difficult types of patients to teach relaxation technique to are patients who have never exercised before, and those who are experiencing high levels of anxiety. The General Relaxation Exercise on page 77 is very definitely indicated for these patients. They must learn what it feels like to contract different areas of the body, and the contrast of "letting go" of the tension. This concept can later be transferred to immediately releasing tension from tight spots on the body with conscious control. Once patients learn this, they can, for example, be sitting at their desks and as soon as they feel their neck or low back area begin to tighten with tension build-up, they can consciously release it by concentrating on the area. This is a practical application of mind and body togetherness, and is very applicable to low-back patients in general, because most have higher than normal levels of tension and anxiety.

Biofeedback is another technique available to teach relaxation. With the electrodes attached to the frontalis muscle, the patient can use both visual and audio feedback to monitor their level of tenseness. Small portable units are available for the patient who finds this method useful, and wishes to practice away from the hospital environment.

Hypnosis (and eventually self-hypnosis) is an excellent method to teach relaxation, especially with patients who have a high eye-roll. For those who can roll their eye-balls up so that a large area of the white of the eye is showing, hypnosis can be a valuable adjunct to their treatment. Attitudes toward exercise programs, habit control, and good health in general can also be established in this manner. Much has been done in this area by Herbert Spiegel, M.D. at Columbia's College of Physicians and Surgeons, and recently his course in clinical hypnosis has been opened to physical therapists.

Yoga and deep breathing exercises are also effective in teaching the patient to achieve mind and body togetherness. Therapists will find that they will be a much better teacher of these techniques if they have already mastered them. Relaxation is a necessary component of every therapeutic exercise program.

Flexibility

Lack of flexibility is one of the leading causes of back pain that is attributable to muscular etiology, mainly because there are several conditions that contribute to increased tension in the muscle or lack of flexibility of the muscle.

The inability to relax sufficiently, to the point where excess tension is eliminated in skeletal muscles, is something we have all experienced at one time or another. Many of us are forced to live and work under stressful conditions, and at the same time have no strenuous physical outlets to dissipate the tensions that naturally build. These tensions cause the muscle to pull away from their physiological resting state, and over a period of time can cause a lack of flexibility in that muscle. As the muscles shorten, an ischemic condition can occur that can eventually cause a painful state, which in turn may precipitate a muscle spasm. Or, when the muscle is in a shortened state, the patient can make any kind of a quick, turn or movement that will suddenly put the muscle on stretch, and cause a tearing of muscle fibers. These fibers can become necrotic because of a lack of blood supply and eventually knot up to form a triggerpoint.

If muscles remain in a shortened state for a long period, they can seriously limit movement around a joint. In time the soft tissue around the joint will calcify, and movement may be lost permanently. It is not unusual to see patients in the clinic who have lost movement of the lumbar vertebra for this very reason. They were either told to keep the back straight to avoid pain, or, decided on their own that it was the movement that was causing the pain, so they simply eliminated it. It is never indicated to teach patients to remain rigid to avoid stress on the back. Rather, they must be taught to move correctly as explained under "Body Movements," otherwise they may spend the rest of their lives rigid, and with an eventual and permanent loss of movement of the lumbar vertebra.

Daily flexibility exercises can remove excess tension from the muscles and prevent this vulnerable state of increased muscle tension and lack of flexibility. The therapist should concentrate on increasing the patient's flexibility before increasing muscle strength for several reasons. First, shortened muscles that are subjected to exercises that add even more tension can easily contribute to muscle spasm by reasons previously mentioned. Secondly, strengthening exercises would strengthen the muscle in a limited range only, and would not help to achieve natural action of the muscle, which is the goal of the exercise. Thirdly, patients can achieve normal movements only by increasing total flexibility, otherwise, they will continue to splint their backs with unnatural contractions, because of limited range, which will add to their lack of mobility rather than increase it. Flexiblity exercises are a necessary prerequisite for all exercise programs, especially for the low-back patient.

Body Posture, Movement and Mechanics

If the therapist has done an adequate job of educating the patient during rehabilitation, or the healthy subject during the beginning stages of the preventive program, the patient should have an easy time understanding and applying the principles of proper body posture, movement, and mechanics. They should know, for instance, the location and function of the iliopsoas muscle and in what position it is contracted (and pulling on the lumbar vertebra) and when it is relaxed. They should thoroughly understand the pelvic tilt and the corresponding muscular and skeletal implications concurrent with an anterior or posterior "tilt." They should understand unequivocally which positions are contraindicated for them, and what circumstances may precipitate an exacerbation of acute low-back pain.

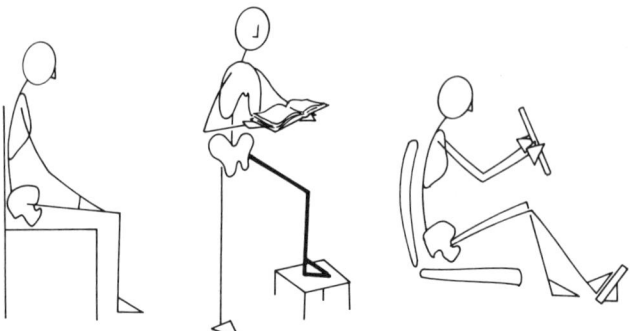

Figure 16. Proper postures during (a) sitting, (b) standing, and (c) driving. Emphasis is on decreasing the lumbar lordosis.

Static Position

Figure 16 shows the correct posture during sitting, standing, and driving. Note that reduction of the lumbar lordosis is the goal of all static positions. In sitting, a straight back chair with firm support for the back and buttocks is best. The feet should easily rest on the floor, and the popiteal area should be at least 3 to 4 in. anterior to the seat of the chair. If the patient is to stand for any length of time, even while brushing teeth and for other ADL activities, he or she should prop one foot (usually the one on the side of pain) up on a stool to reduce the pull of the iliopsoas on the lumbar vertebra. While driving the seat should be far enough forward so that the knees are up higher than the hips in order to reduce iliopsoas tension. A firm seat is also necessary for the buttocks and for reducing the lumbar curve. Many commercial insert seats are available to provide this support; however, in their absence the patient may place a wide board on the seat and a thin pillow behind the back to support the natural lumbar lordosis.

The patient should also be reminded that an anterior tilt of the pelvis is the correct "natural" position for him or her to assume during everyday activities. Direct application of exercises such as the pelvic tilt must be reinforced by informing the patient to assume the standing pelvic tilt while in elevators, trains, against the office wall, or whenever standing is necessary. This type of application of exercise principles into daily living situations not only instills motivation to learn and perform the exercises, but also gives the patient confidence in his or her treatment program and; therefore, in his or her ability to return to a useful and productive life. Every effort must be made by the therapist to continually instill this type of positive reinforcement into the treatment program.

Body Mechanics for Functional Activities

Forty percent of back patients suffer their initial onset of pain during or immediately after lifting or pushing a load. This happens because the average adult loses contact with the idea and the feeling of how his or her body movements have been eliminated from our sedentary lives. Unless a special effort is made, patients do not run, swim, climb hills, or even walk. Without this type of activity it is impossible to keep in touch with our bodies and retain this "mind and body togetherness." Patients, therefore, must be taught to lift, carry, push, and pull objects correctly to prevent back strain during the activity.

Figure 17 demonstrates the reason for holding a load close to the body while lifting or carrying. The muscular stress and compressive force on the disc are increased substantially as the load moves away from the body.

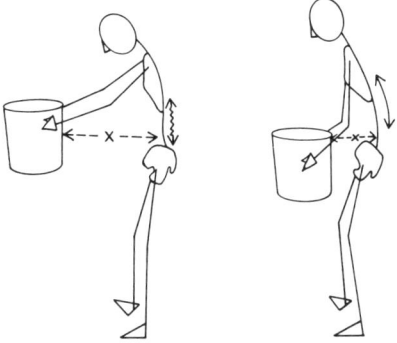

Figure 17. By increasing either the weight of the object (W), or the distance the object is held from the body (x), the muscular stress (M) will increase concurrently. The muscular stress also represents a compressive force on the discs.

Figure 18 shows the proper way to lift. The patient should get as close to the load as possible, take a step forward with one foot, pull in the stomach, and squat down to reach the object. The back should not be kept rigid, but should exhibit a slight curve which will automatically happen when the patient contracts the abdominals. Chin should be tucked throughout. Once the patient has a good grip on the object, he or she begins to exhale slowly while straightening the knees. As the knees straighten, the patient assumes the pelvic tilt by

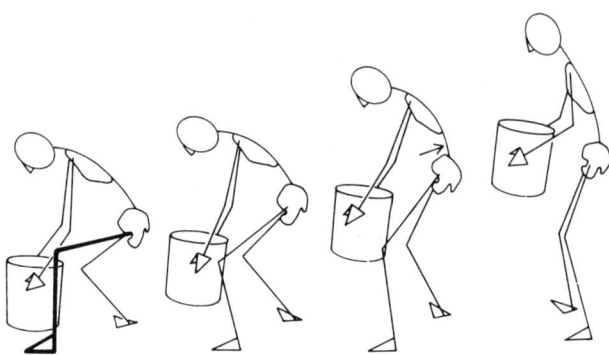

Figure 18.

pinching the buttocks and assumes the upright position. The load remains close to the body throughout. The patient should practice this sequence many times using an empty box or a large plastic ball or any light object, until the movements become natural and easy.

Pushing and pulling become easy when the patient learns to use the force created by the transfer of the entire body weight from one foot to the other. Figure 19a shows the correct way to push. One foot should be in front of the other, and it is the transfer of the patient's weight from the rear foot to the front foot that pushes the object. Note that elbows are bent, chin is tucked, abdominals are contracted, and the patient is exhaling during the working movement. Figure 19b shows the same principles applied to pulling an object. Here the patient drops his or her weight as if he or she is "sitting in a chair," and it is this action that utilizes the entire body weight to pull the object.

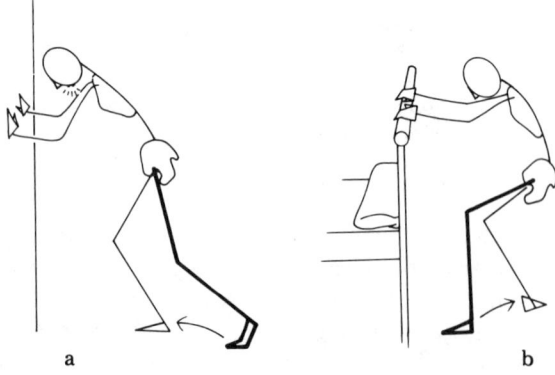

Figure 19.

Considering the three movements of lifting, pulling, and pushing, pulling is the least harmful to the low back, because the rise in intra-abdominal pressure is lowest compared to the other two movements. An object should never be lifted or pushed when it can be pulled. The patient can practice pushing against a wall, and pulling by holding onto a heavy, immovable object. The most important factor to concentrate on during the exercise will be body positions, breathing while doing the work, and transfer of the body weight from one foot to the other.

SUMMARY

Patient education is the goal of the treatment when considering body positioning, movement, and mechanics, regardless of the etiology of the patient's back pain. Patients who are experiencing spasm or post-triggerpoint injection treatment must be taught to avoid aggravating situations, whereas those who suffer from muscular deficiency must learn to move in a protective manner. Those whose pain is of a skeletal etiology must know what positions and movements are contraindicated, and how to safely perform the movements that they will encounter in everyday situations.

All patients must learn relaxation and "mind and body togetherness." Oftentimes, they can be taught concurrently, and the patient can use one to achieve the other. Improving muscle flexibility and strength must always be considered as a protective measure. In addition, patient's must relearn to move naturally, to become reoriented to their bodies and their relationship to space and the environment.

The therapist must make every effort to correlate the patient's exercise program to functional activities the patient will encounter durhis or her specific everyday routine. This will serve three purposes. It will motivate the patient to learn and perform the exercises, prepare the muscles for future demands, and also give the patient the "feel" of the correct way to move during the activity. It will also give the patient confidence in the treatment program and his or her ability to return to normal activities.

No patient should be discharged from the rehabilitation program without knowing his or her entire exercise program and how to apply it. The patient should know whether or not he or she can partake in other athletic endeavors, and which ones are appropriate. The patient should know how to warm-up properly for the sport, and how it can replace his or her individualized program on occasion. The patient should be aware of the anatomy and the mechanics of the back, and which particular positions are contraindicated. The patient should know how to sit, drive, sleep, stand, pick up objects, push, pull, and move properly incorporating all positions that he or she will encounter during his or her daily routine. In this manner, the patient will be best prepared in preventing an episode of low-back pain.

BIBLIOGRAPHY

Belkin, S. C., and Quigley, T. B. (1977). Finding the cause of low back pain. *Medical Times*, July, 1977.

Branton, P. (1969). Behaviour, body mechanics and discomfort. *Ergonomics* 12(2).

Brown, J. R. (1973). Industrial back injury: A look at an old problem. *Ergonomics* 16(4).

Caillet, M. D. (1968). Rehabilitation management of the patient with low back pain. *Mod Treat 5*.

Caillet, R. (1968). *Low Back Pain Syndrome.* 2nd ed. Davis, Philadelphia.

Cairns, D. T., Lynn Mooney, V., and Pace, B. J. (1976). A comprehensive treatment approach to chronic low back pain. *Pain 2*.

Chapman, A. E., and Troup, J. D. G. (1969). The effect of increased maximal strength on the integrated electrical activity of lumbar erectores spinae. *Electromyogr Clin Neurophysiol 9*(2).

Craig, K., Best, A. J. (1977). Perceived control over pain: Individual differences and situational determinants. *Pain 3*.

Davis, P. R., and Troup, J. D. G. (1966). Effects on the trunk of erecting pit props at different working heights. *Ergonomics 9*(6).

Davis, P. R., and Troup, J. D. G. (1974). Pressures in the trunk cavities when pulling, pushing and lifting. *Ergonomics 7*(4).

Farfan, H. F. (1973). *A Mathematical Model of the Soft Tissue Mechanisms of the Lumbar Spine. Mechanical Disorders of the Low Back.* Lea and Febiger, Philadelphia.

Gray, E. R. (1977). Conscious control of motor units in a tonic muscle—The effect of motor unit training. *Am J Phys Med 50*(1).

Grieve, X., and Pheasant, Y. (1976). Myoelectric acitivity, posture and isometric torque in man. *Emg J 16*(1).

Grzesiak, R. C. (1977). Relaxation techniques in treatment of chronic pain. *Arch Phys Med Rehabil 39*(12).

Jayson, M. (Ed). (1976). *The Lumbar Spine and Back Pain.* Sector Publishing Ltd. London.

Jonsson, B. (1970). The functions of the individual muscles in the lumbar part of the spine. *Electromyogr Clin Neurophys 10*(1).

Kraus, H. (1973). Triggerpoints. *NY State Med 73*(11).

Lauder, W. T. (1976). A review of operant conditioning in the treatment of chronic low back pain. *Off J Assoc Rehabil Nurses 1*(2).

Magora, A. (1970). Investigation of the relation between low back pain and occupation. *Industrial Med 39*(12).

Ministry of Labor and Employment, Government of India (1965). Lifting with safety. Industrial Safety and Health Bulletin, Volume VIII, Number 1.

Ministry of Labor Employment and Rehabilitation, Government of India (1967). Seating in Industry. Industrial Safety and Health Bulletin, Volume 10, Number 2.

Nachemson, A. L. (1966). The load on the lumbar discs in different positions of the body. *Clin Orthop 45.*

Nachemson, A. L. (1976). The lumbar spine. An Orthopaedic challenge. *Spine* 1(1).

Nachemson, A. L. (1977). Pathophsiology and treatment of back pain: A critical look at the different types of treatment. *Approaches to Validation of Manipulation Therapy.* A. A. Buerger and J. S. Tubis (Eds.) Thomas, Springfield, IL.

Ortengren, R., and Andersson, G. B. J. (1977). Electromyographic studies of trunk muscles, with special reference to the functional anatomy of the lumbar spine. *Spine* 2(1).

Tichauer, E. R. (1976). Biomechanics sustain occupational. *Industr Eng.*

Troup, J. D. G. (1976). Mechanical factors in spondylolisthesis and spondylolysis. *Clin Orthop,* Number 117.

Wachsler, R. A., and Learner, D. B. (1960). An analysis of some factors influencing seat comfort from General Motors Research Laboratories. *Ergonomics* 3(1).

Weisfeldt, S. C. (1971). Ambulatory approach to the treatment of low back pain. *J Occ Med* 13(8).

Index

A

ADL activities, 15, 36, 141, 154, 163, 176, 186
Ambulation, 19
Anxiety, 10, 183
Assessment
  forms, 42, 43
    muscular, 45, 46, 47, 67
      abdominals, 55
      abdominals and hip flexors, 55
      atrophy, 47
      extensors, upper back, 56
      extensors, lower back, 56
      fibrositis, 45
      flexibility, 47, 56
      gastrocnemius soleus, 57
      hamstrings, 56, 57
      hip flexors, 55, 56
      palpation, 45
      postural, 55
      rectus femoris, 57
      spasm, 45
      specific muscle test, 56
      tensor fascia lata, 57
      triggerpoints, 45
    neurological, 48
      addition tests, 48
      bowstring test, 59
      inspection, 48
      LaSeque sign, 59
      pin prick, bilaterally, 58
      reflexes, 48, 58
      sensation, 48, 58
      sensory disturbances, 48
      straight leg raising, 48, 58, 59
    pain, 50, 51, 139
      activities excluded, 50
      aggravated by, 50
      associated with, 50
      bowel or bladder problems, 50
      completed form, 138
      kind of, 50
      location, 51
      start of, 50
      treatment for, 50
    necessity of, 42
    worksheet, 42, 44

B

Back support, 160
"Ballooned" disc (*See* Herniated nucleus pulposus)
Bed mobility, 150
Bedrest, 180
Biofeedback, 183
Body, movement and mechanics, 15, 164
  continuum of concept, 165
  for functional activities, 187
    lifting, pushing, carrying, 187, 188
  goal of, 165
  loss of, 187
  movement, 165
  muscular deficiency, 167
  patient
    education, 185
      for driving, 186
      for sitting, 185
      for standing, 186
    instruction, 164, 185
  positioning, 147, 165
  posture, 185
  proper approach
    guide, 166
    reinforcement, 176
    teaching, 165, 167
  relationship to space and environment, 189
  weight, transfer of, 188
Bulged disc (*See* Herniated nucleus pulposus)

C

Calcium, 36
Chronic low-back condition, definition, 3
Chronic low-back pain, 1
  sufferers, 1, 2, 5
    biological profile of, 8
    precipitating factors, 7
    preexisting personality profile, 9
    socioeconomic profile, 9
Cold, 19
Concepts, insight into evaluation and treatment, 29
  application of, 29
Conditioning
  sports, 142
  recreational, 142
Contraction, 54
Contracture, 33
  cause of, 33
Contusion, 32
  symptoms of, 32
Conversion hysteria, 16
  anxiety reaction, 16
    functional symptom, 16
  characteristics of, 16, 17
  gain
    primary, 16
    secondary, 16
  phobia, 16
Corset, abdominal support, 177
Current
  surging, 69
  tetanizing, 69

D

Degenerative
  changes, 36
  processes, 34
Depression, 13-14
  cause-and-effect relationship, 14
  prevalence, 14
Disc degeneration, 53
  acute prolapse, 38
    cause of, 38
    symptoms of, 38
    treatment of, 38
  changes, 35
  herniated, material, 39
  processes, 38, 40
  cause of, 38
  sequelae of, 38
  symptomatic, 181
Discogenic/neurological considerations, 38
  acute disc prolapse, 38
  disc degeneration, 38
  herniated nucleus pulposus, 39
  nerve root
    irritation, 39
    pressure, 39
    tension, 39
  segmental instability, 38
Discomfort vs. pain, differentiating between, 142

E

Electrotherapy, 140, 156
Ely's test, 60
Environment
  control over, 27
  restructure of, 27
Estrogen, 36
Etiologies
  of low-back pain, 29, 134
    muscular, 40
    multifaceted, 40
  skeletal
    goal of treatment, 176
    patient attitude to, 176
    preventive program
      "bent over" position, 176
      flexion with rotation, 176
      lifting, 176
      mechanically unloading back, 177
    sports, 176
Examination, clinical, 68
  impression, 68
    differential diagnosis, 68
    initial diagnosis, 68
    rehabilitation goal, 68
  referrals, 68
Exercise, 19, 67, 69, 71, 72, 76
  breathing, 184
    deep, 73
  cool down, 72, 183
  curl-up, 165
  duration, 72
  flexibility, 162
  goal of, 72

how to, 73
isometric, 177
"letting go" of muscle tension, 73, 183
for mobilization, active, 157
preparation
   mental, 163
   physical, 163
preventive program, 182
principles, 186
relaxation, 77-79
strengthening, 141, 185
   abdominals, 177
   hamstrings
      manual resistance, 146
      PRE, 146
stretching, hamstrings, 142, 150
swimming, 182
   increased lordosis, due to, 182
   strokes
      breast, 182
      crawl, 182
      side, 182
traction, natural, 157
types
   abdominal stretching, 113-122
   hamstring stretching, 101-108, 142, 150
   hip abductor strengthening, 95-96
   hip adductor stretching, 130-131
   hip extensor strengthening, 97-100
   hip flexor stretching, 109-112
   limbering, 80-82
   low-back extensor stretching, 88-94
   pelvic tilt, 84-87
   tensor fasciae latae stretching, 127-129
warm up, 72, 183
when not to, 178
when to progress, 146
Exercise program, low-back, application of, 139
Explanation of measurements, 52
   arches, medial, depression or flattening, 53
   chest, 52
      ankylosing spondylitis
         degree of, 52
         sumptoms of, 52
         x-ray findings, 52
   height of shoulders, 52
      cervical lordosis, 52
      dorsal kyphosis, 52
   iliac crests, level of, 52
   leg length, 52
   long-sitting position, 53
Extension, passive, 160

F

Facet dysfunction, 35
   disruption of
      gliding, 35
      weight-bearing functional unit, 35
Feedback
   audio, 184
   bio-, 183
   visual, 184
"Feeling" for natural movements, 165
Femoral stretch, 60
Fibrositis, 45, 54
Fitness, cardiovascular, 155
Flexibility, 33, 47, 141, 181, 182
   as cause of back pain, 184
   examination, 67
   exercises, daily, 185
   lack of, 33, 184
Forces, acting on,
   disc system, 164, 187
   muscular system, 164
   skeletal system, 164
Functional program, 152, 153, 154, 163
   endurance, 152
   power, 152
   speed, 152
   strength, 152
Functional unit, 35

G

Goal, of treatment, 26-27, 134, 163, 189
   long-term, 27, 133, 143
   patient education, 189
   short-term, 27, 133, 163
Gravity
   center of, 168
   use of, 167

H

Hamstring
  contract-relax techniques, 151
  flexibility of, 151
  spasm, 149
    symptoms of, 149
    treatment of, 149
Heat, 19, 161
Hematoma sequelae, 32, 141
Herniated disc (*See* Herniated nucleus pulposus)
Herniated nucleus pulposus, 39, 147
Hip pathology, 39
History, 67, 139
HNP, 180
Home program, 15, 69
Hyperextension, active, 160
Hyperflexion, passive, 160
Hypertension, strains, 35, 38
Hypnosis/self-hypnosis, 184
  attitudes developed during, 184
  high eye roll, 184

I

Ice (ethyl chloride) treatment, 69, 140, 156, 161
  instructions, 75
  massage, 75, 161
  phases, 75-76
Increased muscle tension, 29
Insert seats, commercial, 186
Inspection of
  gluteal crease, 60
  psoriatic lesions, 60
    psoriatic sacroilitis, 60
    spondylitis, 60
  skin changes, 60
Ischial tuberosity, 150

J

Joints
  instability, 36
  lumbosacral, 52
  sacroiliac, 53
    cause of referred pain, 36
    sprains, tests for, 53
    treatment of, 36
  zygapophysial, 35
Junction, lumbosacral, 181

K

Knee jerk, 58
Kraus-Weber test, 46, 55, 144, 156, 163
Kyphosis, 36

L

LaSeque sign, 59
Leg length, discrepancy in, 151
Lesion, extrudal, 37
Ligamentous sprain, 31
  case history, 160
  ligament
    anterior and lateral spinal, 31
    articular, 31
    posterior longitudinal, 31
    supraspinous, 31, 160
  symptoms of, 160
  treatment of, 160
Lithium carbonate (*See* Supportive drugs)
Low-back exercise program, 66
  acute stage, progression from, 66
  patient education, 66
  purpose of, 66
"Low-back transient", 26
Lumbar
  lordosis, 51, 177
  vertebra, loss of, 185

M

Maintenance program, 182
Massage, 19
  friction, 161
  ice, 161
Malingerer, 16
  vs. conversion patient, 17
Manipulation, by patient, 19
Masochism, 9
  definition of, 18
  guilt feelings, 18
  punishment, pain vs. pleasure, 18
Medcolator, 69
Mobilization, active, 157
  exercises for, 158
  to increase mobility of vertebrae, 158
  to stretch trunk muscles in rotary

pattern, 158
Motivation, 155, 158, 163, 189
Movements
  abdominals, 168
  body, 176, 185
    prone back to supine, 170
    prone to hands and knees to
      standing, 173
    side-lying to prone, 170
    sitting to standing, 175
    standing to hands and knees, 174
    standing to sitting in chair, 175
    supine to side-lying, 169
    supine to side sitting, 171
    supine to side sitting to getting
      up from bed, 172
  to check
    extension, 61
    hip range of motion, 62
    knee-kiss position, 62
    lumbar pelvic rhythm, 61
    normal, 142
    rotation, 61
    side bend, 61
  natural, 168
  principles, 168
  rotational, 24
Muscle, 54
  atrophy, 47, 58
  frontalis, 183
    for biofeedback, 183
  iliopsoas, location and function,
    185
  ischemic condition, 184
  loss of length and elasticity, 31
  "pump", 38
  resting length, 29, 71, 72
  spasm, 31, 61, 71, 75, 139-141,
    147, 160, 165, 184
    causes of
      emotional tension, 71
      postural strain, 71
      stress, 71
      sudden change, 71
      trauma, 71
      triggerpoint, 71
  strain, 31
  tenderness, 39, 45, 54
  tension, 163
  tightness, 183
Muscular
  assessment (2)
    abdominals, 55

abdominals and hip flexors, 55
extensors
  upper back, 56
  low back, 56
function test, 55
hip flexors, 55
specific test, 56
assessment (3)
  flexibility, 56
  gastrocnemius soleus, 57
  hamstrings, 56
  hip flexor, 56
  lower back
    with hamstrings, 57
    without hamstrings, 57
  rectus femoris, 57
  tensor fascia lata, 57
/ligamentous considerations, 29
  contracture, 33
  contusion, 32
  flexibility, 33
  hematoma sequelae, 32
  increased muscle tension, 29
  ligamentous sprain, 31
ligament
  anterior and lateral spinal, 31
  articular, 31
  posterior longitudinal, 31
  supraspinous, 31
muscle inbalance, cause of, 31
muscle spasm
  cause of, 31
  definition of, 31
  treatment of, 32
muscle strain, 31
  overuse, 31
  treatment of, 31
muscle weakness, 33
piriformis syndrome, 33
triggerpoint, 32

N

Nerve root
  compression, 58
  irritation, 39, 54
    cause of, 39
  pressure
    cause of, 39
    parethesis vs. paralysis, 39
    symptoms, 39
  tension, 39
    cause of, 39
    test for, 39

Newton's third law, 168
New York Hospital, 3, 11, 14
 Department of Rehabilitation, 3
 Low-Back Exercise Program, 66
New York University Medical Center, 7

O

Occupational therapist, 176
 group sessions with, 176
 role of, 176
Occupational therapy, role of, 27
Osteoarthritis, 36
 cause of, as a degenerative
  process, 36
 treatment of, 36
Osteophytes, 36
Osteoporosis, 35
 cause of, 35-36
 treatment of, 36

P

Pain, 53, 139, 142, 161, 167, 183
 ankylosing spondylitis, 63
 assessment, 62, 67
 chronic low-back, 1, 161
 clinical signs, 2
 cultural determination, 25
 emotional component, 1
 female pelvic organs, 63
 long-standing, 25
 and loss, 21
 low-back, 1
  acute episode, 15, 25
  assessment of, 40
  causes of, 29, 40, 42
  chronic episode, 7
  contradictory treatments, 29
 mechanical, 62
 need for, 21, 24
 precipitating event, 6, 7-8
  childbirth, 6
  falling, 6
  lifting or pushing heavy objects, 6
  traffic accidents, 6
 psychological problems, 63
 psychosomatic, 21
  and depression, 14
 radiating, 63
 referred, 63
 response to, 25
 schematic presentation of (psychosomatic origin), 6
 solution, 42
 spinal metastases, 63
 spine, 63
 TNS in treatment, 19, 161
 tuberculosis, 63
Palpation, 45
Paralyses, 39
Paresthesis, 39
Pathology, primary, 134
Patient
 in-, 153
 low-back, progression of, 25
 out-, 153
 pain-prone, psychological aspects, 7
 positive efforts of, by conditioning, 27
 role, 141
  active, 27
  passive, 27
  unmotivated, 27
Personality profile, preexisting, 8, 9
Physical therapist
 attitude of, 10
  support vs. disinterest, 10
 education of, 26
 emotional support by, 16
 intervention in treatment by, 6
 referral by, 15, 16
 responsibilities of, 14, 26, 66
 role of, 1, 26
  technician or assistant, 26
 treatment by, 2
Physical therapy program
 bracing and supports, 134
 curtailment of activities, 134
 flexibility, 134
 function, 134
 injections, 134
 medication, 134
 muscle strength, 134
 success at New York Hospital, 134
Piriformis syndrome, 33
 cause of, 33
 treatment of, 33
Pool therapy, 19, 156
Positions, curl-up
 axis of motion, 164
 center of gravity, 164
 placement of arms, 164
Posterior ramus, 35
Postlaminectomy
 aching and pulling, 156
 case history of, 155
 movements to be avoided, 156

numbness or weakness, 156
scar tissue, 156
treatment of, 156
Postsurgery, case history, 157
Pressure, intradiscal, 177-180
considerations of, 164-165
curl-up, 165
in relation to position, 164
intra-abdominal, rise in, 189
rest positions, 178
Prevention of back injury for healthy subject, muscular consideration, 181
Preventive medicine, 159
Prolapsed disc (*See* Herniated nucleus pulposus)
Protruded disc (*See* Herniated nucleus pulposus)
Psychiatric assistance, 12
adjunct to, 26
Psychiatrist, 24
role of, 15
Psychosomatic symptom, 10

Q

Quadratus lumborum, contracture of, 151

R

Recreational activities, 153
Referred pain, 34
Reflexes, 48, 58
Rehabilitation efforts
approach, 176
early stages of, 178
interference with, 26
program, discharge from, 189
Relaxation training, 19
general, 70, 79
how to teach, 183
Responsibility of
physician, 66
therapist, 66
Resting physiological state, 163
Ruptured disc (*See* Herniated nucleus pulposus)

S

Scoliosis, 31, 52, 53
curve
"C", 53
compensatory, 53
primary, 53
"S", 53
functional, 35, 53
structural, 35, 53
vertebral rotation, test for, 53
Segmental instability, 38
cause of, 38
hyperextension sprains, because of, 38
Sensation, 48
Sexual intercourse, when to avoid, 166
Skeletal considerations, in initial therapy period, 181
Slipped disc (*See* Herniated nucleus pulposus)
SLR, limited, 150
Specific muscle test, 46, 56
Spinous processes, examination of
alignment, 54
amount of movement, 54
mobility, 54
Spurring, 36
Spondylolisthesis, 34, 53
forward subluxation, 34
sequelae of
disc rupture, 35
nerve root compression, 35
nerve root kinking, 35
strain of supraspinous ligament, 35
Spondylolysis, 33
asymptomatic, 34
disc degeneration, 34
premature, 34
encroachment, extraforaminal and foraminal, 34
vertebral instability, 34
Stimulation, electric, 19
Straight leg raise, bilateral, 53
Strength, muscle, 81
Structural considerations, 33
facet, dysfunction, 35
osteoarthritis, 36
osteoporosis, 35
sacroiliac joint, 36
scoliosis, 35
spondylolisthesis, 34
spondylolysis, 33
Sufferer, acute, 26
Supportive drugs, 16
Symptoms and conditions, most

common, 139
abnormal gait, 136
contracture, 136
fibrositis, 136
improper body mechanics, 136
increased muscle tension, 136
ligamentous sprain, 136
lack of flexibility, 136
limited ROM, 136
loss of functional capacity, 136
loss of normal movement (specific and/or gross), 136
muscle inbalance, 136
muscle spasm, 136
muscle strain, 136
muscle weakness, 136
pain, 136
skeletal strain, 136
triggerpoints, 136
Symptoms, psychosomatic, 22

T

Tension, general, 166
Therapy
  physical, no relief from, 13
  supportive, 5
  ultrasound, 161
Tilt
  awareness of, 146
  pelvis, 157, 177, 185, 187
Traction
  natural, 157
  on the nerve, 39
  spurs, 39
Traditional treatment, failure of, 139
Transcutaneous nerve stimulation (TNS), 19
Transfer of patient
  log rolling, 147
  position, 147
Treatment
  of acute episode, 137
  components
    ADL training, 136
    bracing and supports, 136
    drugs and injections by physicians, 136
    flexibility exercises, 136
    functional program, 136
    limbering, 136
    maintenance-oriented program 136, 137
    mobilization, 136
    muscle strengthening exercises, 136
    other modalities
      electric stimulation, 136
      ice/ethyl chloride, 136
      heat, 136
      massage, 136
      ultrasound, 136
      relaxation training, 136
      TNS, 136
  concepts, 160
  contraindications, 162
  levels of treatment, 160
  postinjection, 69
  program
    guidelines for
      lifestyle, returning to, 133
      motivation, 133
      pain vs. discomfort, 134
      patient education, 133
      reevaluation, 134
  no response to, 140
Tricyclic antidepressants (See Supportive drugs)
Triggerpoint, 32, 45, 141, 161, 165-166
  causes of, 32, 184
    palpation of, 55
    treatment of, 32
  postinjection treatment, 165-166
"Togetherness", mind/body, 183, 184, 187, 189

U

Ultrasound therapy, 161

V

Vertebral instability, 56
  case history, 156
  causes of
    disc degeneration, 156
    trauma, 156
  posterior facet joint, 156

Y

y axis, 180
Yoga, 184

RD768.L28
LaFreniere / The low-back patient : procedures for